Globalization and Health

Understanding Public Health Series

Series editors: Nicki Thorogood and Rosalind Plowman, London School of Hygiene & Tropical Medicine (previous edition edited by Nick Black and Rosalind Raine)

Throughout the world, recognition of the importance of public health to sustainable, safe, and healthy societies is growing. The achievements of public health in nineteenth-century Europe were for much of the twentieth century overshadowed by advances in personal care, in particular in hospital care. Now, with the dawning of a new century, there is increasing understanding of the inevitable limits of individual health care and of the need to complement such services with effective public health strategies. Major improvements in people's health will come from controlling communicable diseases, eradicating environmental hazards, improving people's diets, and enhancing the availability and quality of effective health care. To achieve this, every country needs a cadre of knowledgeable public health practitioners with social, political, and organizational skills to lead and bring about changes at international, national and local levels.

This is one of a series of books that provides a foundation for those wishing to join in and contribute to the twenty-first-century regeneration of public health, helping to put the concerns and perspectives of public health at the heart of policy-making and service provision. While each book stands alone, together they provide a comprehensive account of the three main aims of public health: protecting the public from environmental hazards, improving the health of the public, and ensuring high-quality health services are available to all. Some of the books focus on methods, others on key topics. They have been written by staff at the London School of Hygiene & Tropical Medicine with considerable experience of teaching public health to students from low-, middle-, and high-income countries. Much of the material has been developed and tested with postgraduate students both in face-to-face teaching and through distance learning.

The books are designed for self-directed learning. Each chapter has explicit learning objectives, key terms are highlighted, and the text contains many activities to enable the reader to test their own understanding of the ideas and material covered. Written in a clear and accessible style, the series will be essential reading for students taking postgraduate courses in public health and will also be of interest to public health practitioners and policy-makers.

Titles in the series

Analytical models for decision making: Colin Sanderson and Reinhold Gruen
Conflict and health: Natasha Howard, Egbert Sondorp and Annemarie Ter Veen (eds.)
Controlling communicable disease: Norman Noah
Economic analysis for management and policy: Stephen Jan, Lilani Kumaranayake, Jenny Roberts, Kara Hanson and Kate Archibald
Economic evaluation: Julia Fox-Rushby and John Cairns (eds.)
Environmental epidemiology: Paul Wilkinson (ed.)
Environmental health policy: Megan Landon and Tony Fletcher
Financial management in health services: Reinhold Gruen and Anne Howarth
Health care evaluation: Sarah Smith, Don Sinclair, Rosalind Raine and Barnaby Reeves
Health promotion theory, Second Edition: Liza Cragg, Maggie Davies and Wendy Macdowall (eds.)
Introduction to epidemiology, Second Edition: Ilona Carneiro and Natasha Howard
Introduction to health economics, Second Edition: Lorna Guinness and Virginia Wiseman (eds.)
Issues in public health, Second Edition: Fiona Sim and Martin McKee (eds.)
Making health policy, Second Edition: Kent Buse, Nicholas Mays and Gill Walt
Managing health services: Nick Goodwin, Reinhold Gruen and Valerie Iles
Medical anthropology: Robert Pool and Wenzel Geissler
Principles of social research, Second Edition: Mary Alison Durand and Tracey Chantler (eds.)
Public health in history: Virginia Berridge, Martin Gorsky and Alex Mold
Sexual health: A public health perspective: Kay Wellings, Kirstin Mitchell and Martine Collumbien (eds.)
Understanding health services: Nick Black and Reinhold Gruen

Forthcoming titles

Environment, health and sustainable development, Second Edition: Emma Hutchinson and Sari Kovats
Health promotion practice, Second Edition: Will Nutland and Liza Cragg (eds.)

Globalization and Health

Second edition

Edited by Johanna Hanefeld

 Open University Press

Open University Press
McGraw-Hill Education
McGraw-Hill House
Shoppenhangers Road
Maidenhead
Berkshire
England
SL6 2QL

email: enquiries@openup.co.uk
world wide web: www.openup.co.uk

and Two Penn Plaza, New York, NY 10121-2289, USA

First published 2015

A catalogue record of this book is available from the British Library

ISBN-13: 978-0-33-526408-7 (pb)
ISBN-10: 0-33-526408-5 (pb)
eISBN: 978-0-33-526409-4

Library of Congress Cataloging-in-Publication Data
CIP data applied for

Typesetting and e-book compilations by
RefineCatch Limited, Bungay, Suffolk

Fictitious names of companies, products, people, characters and/or data that may be used herein (in case studies or in examples) are not intended to represent any real individual, company, product or event.

Printed and bound by CPI Group (UK) Ltd, Croydon, CR0 4YY

Praise for this book

"This is a vital book which addresses the public health implications of accelerating globalisation. It shows with forensic clarity the dire impact neoliberal economics and burgeoning corporate power is having on individual, collective and planetary health. At the same time it holds out the hope that civil society can respond to this challenge and develop governance systems which ensure that the currently predominant free-market logic is reversed and people are once more put firmly before profits. Study it; learn from it; make a difference."

Gerard Hastings, University of Stirling, UK, and the Open University

"This book provides a clear introduction to how globalization is shaping our health and the determinants of health. The authors not only introduce us to the growing field of global health, but also provide some concrete evidence of driving factors, the key players and the impact on our daily lives. It should be a reference book for public health students, public health practitioners, as well as for policy makers. After I read this book I really realized that I live in a global village with all the consequences. Congratulations, it is a really great book."

Asnawi Abdullah, Faculty of Public Health,
University Muhammadiyah Aceh, Indonesia

Contents

List of figures, tables, and boxes

Figures

Tables

Boxes

List of contributors

Joan Busfield is a Professor in the Department of Sociology at the University of Essex.

Dr Nick Drager, Former Director of the Department of Ethics, Equity, Trade and Human Rights and Senior Adviser in the Strategy Unit, Office of the Director-General at the World Health Organization, is now Honorary Professor of Global Health Policy at the London School of Hygiene & Tropical Medicine.

Dr Andy Guise is a Research Fellow at the University of California San Diego and London School of Hygiene & Tropical Medicine.

Dr Johanna Hanefeld is Lecturer in Health Systems Economics and the Director of the Anthropology, Politics and Policy Group at the London School of Hygiene & Tropical Medicine.

Dr Ben Hawkins is a political scientist studying the influence of interests and evidence on the policy process. He is a Lecturer in the Department of Global Health and Development at the London School of Hygiene & Tropical Medicine.

Kelley Lee is Tier 1 Canada Research Chair in Global Health, Faculty of Health Sciences at Simon Fraser University, British Columbia, Canada and Honorary Professor of Global Health Policy, London School of Hygiene & Tropical Medicine.

Dr Marco Liverani is a Lecturer in the Department of Global Health and Development, London School of Hygiene & Tropical Medicine.

Tony McMichael was a Professor of Population Health at the Australian National University and from 1994-2001 was Professor of Epidemiology at the London School of Hygiene & Tropical Medicine. He sadly died in September 2014, as this book was going to press.

Neil Pearce is Professor of Epidemiology and Biostatistics and Director of the Centre for Global NCDs at the London School of Hygiene & Tropical Medicine.

Richard Smith is Professor of Health System Economics and Dean of Faculty of Public Health & Policy, London School of Hygiene & Tropical Medicine.

Dr Neil Spicer is a Lecturer in Global Health Policy at the London School of Hygiene & Tropical Medicine.

Professor Carolyn Stephens is Executive Director of the Amazonia-Yungas Observatory for Biodiversity, Indigenous Health & Equity. She holds joint appointments with UCL Institute of Health Equity/London School of Hygiene & Tropical Medicine and Facultad de Medicina, Universidad Nacional de Tucumán, Argentina.

Dr Preslava Stoeva is a Lecturer in the Department of Global Health and Development and Course Director of the MSc Global Health Policy (DL) at the London School of Hygiene & Tropical Medicine.

Dr Helen Walls is a Research Fellow in Nutrition and Health with the London School of Hygiene & Tropical Medicine and the Leverhulme Centre for Integrative Research on Agriculture and Health.

Acknowledgements

Open University Press and the London School of Hygiene & Tropical Medicine have made every effort to obtain permission from copyright holders to reproduce material in this book and to acknowledge these sources correctly. Any omissions brought to our attention will be remedied in future editions.

We would like to express our grateful thanks to the copyright holders for granting permission to reproduce material in this book from the following sources:

ITU World Telecommunication/ICT Indicators Database (Figure 1.2)

UN Conference on Trade and Development (Figure 1.3)

OECD/International Transport Forum (Table 7)

Milton Jung, Photo (http://upload.wikimedia.org/wikipedia/commons/7/75/Favela_do_Moinho_Brazil_Slums.jpg)

The Economist (Figure 3.1)

World Bank (Organization Chart of the World Bank)

http://siteresources.worldbank.org/EXTABOUTUS/Resources/bank.pdf

OECD (Figure 3.3)

World Bank (Figure 3.5)

World Bank (Figure 3.6)

World Bank (Figure 3.7)

WTO (Structure of the World Trade Organization)

BMJ (Four stages of the tobacco epidemic)

Edward Arnold (Respiratory tuberculosis death rates, England and Wales, 1838–1970)

Elsevier (Cause of death across countries, by World Bank income group, 2008)

Sheridan Press (Proportion of major food groups advertised to children, by country)

Taylor and Francis (Fragile food supply chains: reacting to risks)

World Resources Institute (World Greenhouse Gas Emissions by Sector and Activity)

World Resources Institute (Carbon Emissions by country 2007 and projected 2030)

World Resources Institute (Impacts of climate change on agricultural output)

World Resources Institute (Water Stress by Country)

UNEP/GRID-Sioux Falls (Estimates of the human overloading of the biocapacity of the Earth)

World Resources Institute (Constituents of well-being)

World Health Organization (Policies and strategies to promote social equity in health)

Introduction to globalization and health

1

Johanna Hanefeld and Kelley Lee

Overview

This chapter provides an introduction to globalization and health and the growing field of global health. It begins by defining the often used, yet highly debated, term 'globalization'. This is accompanied by a conceptual framework for understanding its distinct features. A discussion of why globalization is happening – the key technological, economic, and political drivers – then follows. The chapter concludes with a discussion of the shift from international to global health arising as a result of globalization, and some of the recent trends within this field.

Learning objectives

After working through this chapter, you will be able to:

- define the concepts of global change and globalization, and discuss the key debates surrounding them
- describe a conceptual framework for understanding the connection between globalization and health
- describe the various drivers and forms of global change (e.g. environmental, economic)

Key terms

Dimensions of global change: The three types of changes – spatial, temporal, and cognitive – that characterize globalization.

Global health: A health issue where the determinants or outcomes are not contained by the territorial boundaries of states, and thus may be beyond the capacity of individual countries to address them through domestic institutions alone.

Globalization: A set of global processes that are intensifying the interconnected nature of human interaction across economic, political, cultural, and environmental spheres.

What does globalization mean?

It is easy to become overwhelmed by the subject of globalization given widespread interest among policy-makers, the business community, academia, mass media, and the general public. The term has generated a burgeoning literature that threatens to swamp even the most enthusiastic reader. Nor is this literature cohesive in content or perspective. Newcomers to the field must immediately recognize that the term 'globalization' is highly contested and its precise meaning is under debate. There are four main points of debate within the vast globalization literature:

- Is globalization actually happening or not? Is globalization actually new? Is it happening to everyone?
- What are the reasons behind what is happening? What are the causes or drivers?
- What is the time-frame for what is happening? Is it a recent phenomenon or does it have historical roots?
- Is the impact of globalization positive or negative? Is it different for different populations in different settings?

Certainly many people are talking about globalization, many of whom have strong and often opposing views about the subject. The task of this chapter, therefore, is not simply to present you with the 'facts'. Many of these so-called 'facts' are contested, depending on who you are, what values you hold, how rich you happen to be, and so on. We cannot provide you with an easy resolution of these conflicting views. What you can be is informed about what kinds of debates are taking place and the different perspectives being put forth on various issues. It will then be up to you to think about your own lives, weigh up the evidence, sort through different value systems, and decide what you think about these issues.

We can begin by attempting to define globalization more clearly. There are many different definitions of globalization available. Here are a few examples of quite diverse definitions of globalization:

> By globalization we simply mean the process of increasing interconnectedness between societies such that events in one part of the world more and more have effects on peoples and societies far away.
>
> (Baylis et al. 2008)

> what we in the Third World have for several centuries called colonization.
>
> (Khor 1995)

> a stretching of social, political and economic activities across frontiers such that events, decisions and activities in one region of the world can come to have significance for individuals and communities in distant regions of the globe.
>
> (Held et al. 1999)

Khor (1995), from the non-governmental organization (NGO) Third World Network, is critical, seeing globalization as an extension of colonization of the developing world. Held et al. (1999) see globalization as a more complex set of processes, focusing on how events, decisions, and activities in one part of the world can have consequences in other parts of the world. This is often referred to as a greater interdependence or interrelatedness of the world.

Definitions of globalization and efforts to define it were prominent in the academic and popular debates during the 1990s. Over the past ten years there has been a shift, with most commentators and analysts now concurring with Jenkins (2004) that globalization is the key social and economic trend over the past decades (Kruk 2012).

Activity 1.1

Select a national newspaper published in your country that you can access daily in hard copy or online. For one week scan and clip any stories and articles using the words 'global' or 'globalization'. Make a file of your clippings or print out the articles.

Is globalization defined and if so, how? Make a note of the various definitions of globalization used. Where it is not defined, is a definition implied? If possible, identify who holds the definition – government official, corporate executive, NGO worker, and so on. What aspect of globalization does each story focus upon (e.g. economic, environmental, social)? Do the articles identify any winners and losers from globalization? Try to decide if each story presents a positive or negative perspective on globalization.

A conceptual framework for understanding globalization and health

This book argues that despite the range of views on globalization presented in the literature, there are certain common features and characteristics that are shared. If we put aside the rather tangled mess of definitions found in the existing literature, we could begin by thinking about what is distinct. How might we decide if the world is changing, or whether any change represents a radical break with the past? What changes are we experiencing around us?

One framework for understanding globalization is to focus on three dimensions of global change: spatial, temporal, and cognitive. First, globalization is leading to changes to human societies along the *spatial dimension*. Globalization is creating changes to how we perceive and experience physical or territorial space. This is perhaps the easiest aspect of globalization for us to grasp.

Spatial changes

The physical world, of course, is the same size as it has always been. But what is different is how we, as human beings, interact with that space: how we move across territorial space, how we define and use space, and how we interact across physical distances is being changed as a consequence of globalization.

Foremost is the increase in population mobility. Not much more than one generation ago, most people stayed near to where they were born and grew up. Travel was rare, expensive, and involved short distances. Since the 1980s, for many people, it has become more affordable to travel over long distances. Travel might be temporary, such as for business, study or due to unexpected displacement. Or travel can be longer term, such as when people migrate to settle elsewhere more permanently. Today, we are a generation on the move like never before, and trends in increasing population mobility are expected to continue. The following statistics illustrate this:

- In 2013, according to the UN, 232 million people, or 3.2 per cent of the world's population, were international migrants, compared with 2.9 per cent (154 million) in 1990.
- The data show that South–South migration is as common as South–North migration. In 2013, about 82.3 million international migrants who were born in the South were living

in a different country in the South compared with 81.9 million international migrants originating in the South and living in the North.

- The UN High Commissioner for Refugees estimates that the total number of refugees and others of concern to the organization (such as asylum seekers and internally displaced persons) reached 45.2 million in 2013, a substantial increase from 1.4 million in 1961.
- Data from the World Tourism Organization show that total international arrivals worldwide reached 1.087 billion in 2013. Europe led growth in absolute terms with an increase of 5 per cent to reach a total of 563 million arrivals. The strongest growth, however, was in Asia and the Pacific, where the number of arrivals grew by more than 6 per cent.

As we move around the world, we bring animals (including microbes) and plants with us, either deliberately or unintentionally. This may occur on an individual scale, such as when we harbour a cold or influenza virus, or sometimes something far worse. This was how the outbreak of H1N1, also referred to as 'swine flu', spread rapidly around the world from where it was first isolated in Mexico. Similarly, six years earlier SARS spread via air travel from China to 30 countries (resulting in a total of 8098 cases and 774 deaths). The movement of life forms can also occur on a larger scale, such as when ships on one side of the world fill up their ballasts with sea water, along with all sorts of marine life, and empty that water at their destination in another part of the world. Mass movement of life forms also occurs through flourishing global economic and trade relations. The introduction of cash crops in many parts of the world has displaced many native plant species. Mass production in larger and larger farms has reduced the varieties of certain crops grown, such as corn, wheat, and potatoes. It is feared that the increased growing of genetically modified organisms (GMOs) will accelerate this trend.

The spatial dimension of global change is thus one key aspect of how we can understand globalization. Globalization as spatial change has been described as:

> growth of 'supraterritorial' relations between people . . . a far-reaching change in the nature of social space.
>
> (Scholte 2000)

> processes through which sovereign national states are criss-crossed and undermined by transnational actors.
>
> (Beck 1999)

> intensification of worldwide social relations which link distant localities in such a way that local happenings are shaped by events occurring many miles away and vice versa.
>
> (Giddens 1990)

Temporal change

The second dimension of global change is *temporal* – how we perceive and experience time. The link between space and time is a close one. We are able to move about more quickly and across greater distances because of available technologies such as jet airliners and high-speed trains. Alternatively, we may not need to cross physical distances any more to interact with other people because we can use other forms of communication, notably the Internet, that are quicker and more accessible than ever before. The experience of an accelerated time-frame can be seen in the following example from medical research. Decoding of genetic sequencing has relied heavily on the computing capacity of prevailing technologies. During the 1970s, it took two months to sequence 150 nucleotides, the letters that spell out a gene. It took 1000 scientists around ten years to decode the first yeast genome. However, due to greater computer processing speeds, today the same process takes hours instead of years.

However, anyone with an e-mail address will know that globalization may or may not mean a net saving in time. Because of our capacity to interact more readily, we may do so more frequently (and spend more time responding to others). Or we might spend more time travelling because of the availability of cheap flights. In other ways, life seems to have slowed down – dealing with large bureaucracies, negotiating the automated telephone options of a large organization, or finding ourselves stuck on increasingly congested roads. More accurately, therefore, globalization is changing our relationship with time. We are spending our time differently compared with a generation ago. For a lucky few who are enjoying the fruits of globalization, leisure time may increase relative to working hours. For many, the pressures of life in a 'post-industrial society' can mean juggling an increasing number of commitments, while for others, the insecurities of work or unemployment mean a very different set of pressures. Here are some quotes from writers who describe the temporal dimension of global change:

> we have been experiencing, these last two decades, an intense phase of time–space compression that has had a disorienting and disruptive impact.
>
> (Harvey 1989)

> a growing magnitude or intensity of global flows.
>
> (Held and McGrew 2000)

> global transactions . . . can extend anywhere in the world at the same time and can unite locations anywhere in effectively no time.
>
> (Scholte 2000)

The field of health has benefited from some of the temporal change, including increased travel and communication technology, which has allowed greater research collaboration and rapid advances in science and medicine that would be hard to imagine without them. On the other hand, the changes in working patterns described may affect health negatively.

Cognitive change

The third dimension of change associated with globalization is *cognitive*. This refers to how globalization is changing what we think about ourselves and the world around us. Some of the main agents of cognitive change are the mass media, advertising agencies, consultancy firms, research and educational institutions, religious groups, and political parties. The thought processes being influenced by their activities include cultural values, beliefs, ideologies, policies, and knowledge.

Among these, perhaps the most ubiquitous in contemporary societies is the mass media, which, in their restructuring and influence, have become global. Until the 1980s, print and broadcast media in most countries were national in scope. There has been trade in books, films, music and television programmes across countries for decades, but broadcasting and publishing industries remained largely domestic in ownership and regulation. Since the 1980s, there has been a technological convergence in modes of communications, and many argue a corresponding convergence in the content of the messages they convey. This has been the result of widespread deregulation and privatization of the telecommunications sector, initially in the USA and Europe, and more recently in middle- and low-income countries.

For the past decade, the Internet has been at the centre of changes in how media are produced and consumed. Several characteristics of the global media landscape have shaped how people access and consume news, which in turn determines their impact on how we perceive the world. First among these has been a consolidation of media ownership. Table 1.1 shows the extent of concentration in media ownership by some of the largest transnational companies and their subsidiaries. With many national media outlets

Table 1.1 Global media giants and their subsidiaries, 2012

News Corporation	Production: Twentieth Century Fox, Blue Sky Studios, Fox Searchlight Pictures
	Broadcasting: FOX News, National Geographic's cable, British Sky Broadcasting, STAR TV (Asia)
	Books: HarperCollins General Book Group, Regan Books, Amistad Press, William Morrow & Co., Avon Books
	Print media: *New York Post* (USA), *The Times* (UK), *The Sun* (UK), *The Australian* (Australia), *The Daily Telegraph* (Australia), *The Herald Sun* (Australia), *The Advertiser* (Australia)
Bertelsmann	Internet: AOL Europe (partial ownership), Barnesandnoble.com (partial ownership with Barnes and Noble), CDNow, Lycos Europe (partial ownership), Napster (partial stake)
	Broadcasting: UFA Film & TV Production (Germany), Trebitsch Production (Germany), Delux Productions (Luxembourg), Cinevideo (Canada), Holland, Media House (Netherlands), First Choice (UK); 16 TV stations in Germany, France, Luxembourg, the Netherlands, Belgium, England, Poland, and Hungary
	Books: Ballantine Publishing Group, Bantam Doubleday Dell, Bertelsmann Publishing Group
Viacom	Networks: CBS, UPN, MTV Network, MTV, Nickelodeon, Nick at Nite, TV Land, CMT, TNN, VH, Noggin (joint venture with Children's Television Workshop), Showtime Networks, Showtime
	Books: The Free Press, MTV Books, Nickelodeon Books, Simon & Schuster, Pocket Books, Scribner, Touchstone.
	Production and Distribution: Paramount Pictures, MTV Films, Nickelodeon Movies
The Walt Disney Company	Production: Walt Disney Pictures, Touchstone Pictures, Hollywood Pictures, Caravan Pictures, Miramax Films, Buena Vista Home Entertainment, Buena Vista
	Networks: ABC, The Disney Channel, SoapNet, ESPN (partial ownership with Hearst), A&E (partial ownership with Hearst and GE), The History Channel (partial ownership with Hearst and GE), Lifetime (partial ownership with Hearst), E! (partial ownership with Comcast, MediaOne and Liberty Media); 10 TV stations.
	Television Production/Distribution: Buena Vista Television, Touchstone Television, Walt Disney Television, Animation

	Books: Walt Disney Company Book Publishing, Hyperion Books, Talk/Miramax Books
AOL TimeWarner	Networks: WB Television Network, HBO, Cinemaxx, Time Warner Sports, Comedy Central (50:50-owned with Viacom), CNN, CNN/fn, CNN/SI, CNN Headline News, TBS,TNT, Cartoon Network, Turner Classic Movies, Court TV (partial ownership)
	Production/Distribution: HBO Independent Productions, New Line Television, Turner Original Productions, Warner Brothers Television, Warner Brothers, Animation, AOL, CompuServe, Netscape, Warner Brothers Studios, Castle Rock Entertainment, New Line Cinema, Fine Line Features
Sony	Production/Distribution: Columbia TriStar Domestic Television, Columbia TriStar International Television, Sony Pictures Family Entertainment, Telemundo Group (partial ownership)
	Cable: Sony Entertainment Television (India, Latin America), Game Show Network (jointly owned with Liberty Digital), HBO Asia (partial ownership), SET Asia (partial ownership), Cinemax Asia (partial ownership), HBO Ole, Latin America (partial ownership), Cinemax, Latin America (partial ownership), E! Entertainment Television, Latin America (partial ownership), The Movie Channel, Middle East (partial ownership), Showtime, Australia (partial ownership), Encore, Australia (partial ownership), Sky Cinema, Japan (partial ownership)
	Production/Distribution: Sony Pictures Entertainment, Columbia Pictures, Sony Pictures Classics, Screen Gems, TriStar Pictures, Columbia TriStar Films (UK), Columbia TriStar Film Distributors, Sony Pictures Imageworks (animation), Sony Pictures Studios, Sony Pictures Digital Entertainment, Sony Online Entertainment, Sony Computer Entertainment (computer games, PlayStation).

in different countries now belonging to large transnational companies, much of the news consumed is produced by one of these global media actors, with coverage in a number of countries often relying on the same sources. Consolidation of media ownership has also made it harder for smaller news outlets or individual newspapers to compete financially in terms of advertising or reach of their coverage and correspondents.

In addition, the Internet company Google has surpassed more traditional media players as the largest media company worldwide (see Figure 1.1). This is indicative of wider trends, with the Internet serving as the major source of news for an increasing number of

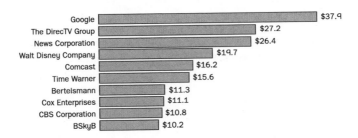

Figure 1.1 The top 10 global media owners and their revenue, 2011 (US$ billions)

Source: ZenithOptimedia

people. A further aspect of this trend is the extent to which social media sites such as Facebook and Twitter have become sources of news for people and also allow people connected to these media to generate content. This further changes the structure and practice of media globally and also allows for closer connection between people across the globe, often without stories being mediated by a journalist or editor.

Entertainment or public broadcasting corporations such as the BBC or CBC are also increasingly in competition with outlets broadcasting directly via the Internet. These changes in communication and media, resulting from the development of online and mobile technology, enable more immediate and greater exchanges between people living in different countries or continents. Given the sheer size of these companies and their ability to entertain, inform, and sell to us, it is perhaps not surprising that people believe they have the power to influence our thoughts. The extent and manner of communication together with media ownership (i.e. who controls the content of information we receive) are argued by some as having had an impact on our thought processes and can be seen as cognitive influence of globalization.

The following are some descriptions of the cognitive dimension of global change:

> the compression of the world and the intensification of consciousness of the world as a whole.
>
> (Robertson 1992)

> McWorld's homogenization is likely to . . . [lead to] the triumph of commerce and its markets and to give to those who control information, communication, and entertainment ultimate control over human destiny.
>
> (Barber 1992)

> We cannot hope to preserve every culture in the world just as it is. And we cannot want a culture to be preserved if it lacks the internal will and cohesion to do so itself. As with species, cultures spawning, evolving and dying is part of evolution. But what is going on today, thanks to globalization, is turbo-evolution.
>
> (Friedman 1999)

For health, this greater interconnectedness and cognitive change can be seen for example in greater solidarity around health issues, such as the treatment access campaigns relating to HIV and AIDS. The cognitive changes also have effects on mental health, which may also be related to other aspects of globalization such as increasing urbanization and changing social roles (see also Chapter 2).

To summarize thus far, it is important to recognize that globalization is probably best understood as a complex set of processes, drivers, and consequences that we need to untangle in order to understand their health impacts. While there tends to be a strong focus on economic globalization – the global economy, capital flows, market restructuring, foreign investment, and so on – this is only one face of globalization. Globalization affects many aspects of our lives, including health, both directly and indirectly. The different dimensions of globalization have already pointed to some of these, including the greater movement of people and pathogens, greater knowledge exchange across physical borders leading to scientific advances, increased solidarity around health issues. This is in addition to challenges in mental and physical health and well-being, as the social patterns of our lives have changed.

Activity 1.2

Refer to your newspaper articles on globalization collected in Activity 1.1. Review the stories again and this time see if you can identify whether they refer to spatial, temporal or cognitive globalization. Do they discuss economic, political, cultural or environmental change?

The technologies behind globalization

Technology is frequently seen as the key driver of global change. It is the most visible manifestation of the changes around us, enabling us to do the things we associate with globalization. Two key technological innovations – information and transportation technology – are further discussed here.

Information technology as a key driver of globalization

As we have seen in the discussion of the cognitive dimension of globalization, information technology has been critical to the kinds of changes associated with globalization.

The nineteenth century saw the introduction of telegraphy, followed by radio and telephony in the early twentieth century. Over the next one hundred years, further enormous leaps in technological development were witnessed: television, undersea cables, satellites, personal computers, facsimile, mobile telephones, and the Internet to name a few. Figure 1.2 illustrates the steep rise in the use of the Internet over the past decade. The two graphs not only highlight that two-thirds of people in the developed world now use the Internet regularly, they also show the extent to which access to the Internet and the opportunities this access provides are unequally distributed. It highlights the extent to which globalization affects different populations differently.

One major reason for this exponential growth in use has been falling costs. This is demonstrated most dramatically by the cost of telephone calls over time. For example, in 1930, it would have cost US$245 to make a three-minute call from London to New York, compared with US$3 in 1990. In 2003, this same telephone call cost US$1, whereas by 2013 such a call will have been possible at a fraction of this cost.

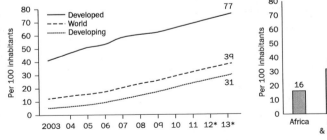
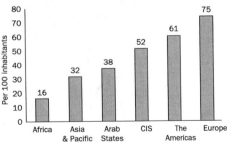

Figure 1.2 Estimated number of Internet users by development level, 2003–13, and by region, 2013

Source: ITU World Communications/ICT Indicators database

Note: *Estimate.

Transportation technology as a driver of global change

Technological developments have also been a key driver of temporal change. With new technologies, we can do lots of things faster.

Processors are not only used in personal computers. They are important for computers used in all sorts of settings, such as by stock exchanges for worldwide financial trading, by banks to carry out electronic transactions, by airlines to book and coordinate flights and passengers, by retailers to manage stock and other logistics, by the mass media to create and transmit programmes, by telecom companies for sending and receiving information. The increased speed of processors has had widespread uses in society, enabling us to do a whole range of things much faster.

Long-haul flights, bullet trains, and supertankers all enable us to move ourselves and our possessions farther and more frequently than ever before. This is because the cost of transport has declined significantly. Figure 1.3 shows the increase in trade and in maritime transport of merchandise; 80 per cent of the world's traded merchandise is transported by sea (UNCTAD 2013). The data in the figure show that maritime trade has more than doubled since 1980. Larger capacity ships, more efficient engines, fuel costs, and greater market competition have all made it financially cheaper to ship freight by sea.

Similarly for air transport, the financial cost per passenger mile has declined roughly six-fold from US$0.68 to US$0.11 due to technological developments in airplane design and size, economies of scale, and keener market competition (UNDP 1999). The number of passengers passing through the world's busiest airport, Atlanta – almost one hundred

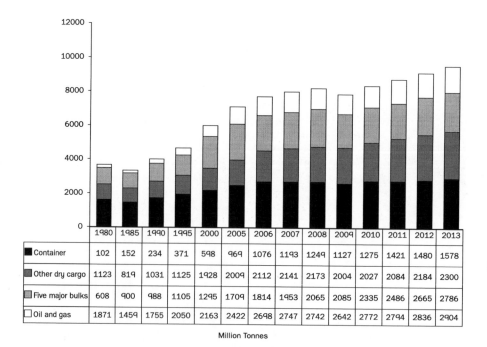

	1980	1985	1990	1995	2000	2005	2006	2007	2008	2009	2010	2011	2012	2013
Container	102	152	234	371	598	969	1076	1193	1249	1127	1275	1421	1480	1578
Other dry cargo	1123	819	1031	1125	1928	2009	2112	2141	2173	2004	2027	2084	2184	2300
Five major bulks	608	900	988	1105	1295	1709	1814	1953	2065	2085	2335	2486	2665	2786
Oil and gas	1871	1459	1755	2050	2163	2422	2698	2747	2742	2642	2772	2794	2836	2904

Million Tonnes

Figure 1.3 Rise in transport of different types of merchandise

Source: UNCTAD Review of Maritime Transport, various issues. For 2006–2013, the breakdown by type of dry cargo is based on Clarkson Research Services' Shipping Review and Outlook, various issues, Data for 2013 are based on a forecast by Clarkson Research Services (2013a)

Table 1.2 The ten busiest airports in the world, 2011

Airport	Code	Total passengers (millions)	Per cent change 2011/10
Atlanta	ATL	92.3	3.4
Beijing	PEK	77.4	4.7
London	LHR	69.4	5.0
Chicago	ORD	66.6	−0.5
Tokyo	HND	62.2	−2.9
Los Angeles	LAX	61.8	4.8
Paris	CDG	60.9	4.8
Dallas	DFW	57.8	1.6
Frankfurt	FRA	56.4	6.5
Hong Kong	HKG	53.3	5.9

Source: OECD (2012).

million – highlights this (Table 1.2). The increased mobility (temporal change) of course also affects our relationship to space (the spatial dimension of globalization) as well as our cognition – that is, how we relate to others. It also enables the greater and more rapid spread of diseases, which is explored further in Chapter 12.

It is important to note the associated environmental costs from increased use of transport technologies (OECD 2008). There is also potentially serious damage from oil spills due to increased sea traffic. These 'costs' are created yet largely omitted from any assessment of the price of globalization. Moreover, such costs are borne inequitably.

 Activity 1.3

Make a list of transportation and communication technologies that you use in your work and private life. Think about how the way you would work and live without these.

Do the technologies allow you to do things differently? Do the technologies allow you to interact with people across time and distance more readily? Would you be able to learn and work in the way you do without them?

The field of global health

As a result of the changes associated with globalization, and their effects on health, global health has increasingly been articulated as a field of study, research, and action. This is distinct from international health, which focuses more narrowly on issues between countries and has a strong historic association with the field of international development, often referring to health interventions undertaken in low- and middle-income countries (Bozorgmehr 2010). While definitions of global health vary and are contested, there is consensus that it focuses on more than health issues between territorially discrete states, addressing health determinants and outcomes that are trans-boundary (i.e.

crossing, transcending or redefining territorial space). Consequently, understanding global health concerns is also often described as requiring multidisciplinary approaches, going beyond more narrowly defined fields of clinical medicine and public health, to include a broader array of disciplines such as economics, law, and political science. Applying knowledge about global health, in turn, requires diverse (and sometimes new) actors beyond the state, such as civil society organizations and private philanthropic foundations (Koplan et al. 2009). Frenk and colleagues (2013) state that global health is:

> defined by two key elements: its level of analysis, which involves the entire population of the world, and the relationship of interdependence that bind together the units of social organization that make up the global population (e.g. nation states, private organizations, ethnic groups, and civil society movements).

The structure, characteristics, and governance of global health form the focus of the next chapter of this book.

Summary

Global health has emerged rapidly as a field of study but is still being refined in terms of clearer definition and conceptualization. At the heart of global health are changes being brought about by globalization, an often contested term to describe a greater intensity and extent of people, other life forms, capital, knowledge and ideas moving across national boundaries. These changes affect every aspect of our lives, including our health and the determinants of health, which often lie outside the areas we associate with medicine or health. This book explores the actors that shape global health, including private companies, foundations, civil society organizations, and multilateral organizations. It looks at how globalization is shaping health, even in areas such as trade and investment, migration and the environment; and it examines key areas of health where the impact of globalization is felt, such as communicable and non-communicable diseases. We begin this exploration of the link between globalization and health through considering social change linked to globalization (Chapter 2). The book then moves on to introduce the global economy and impacts on health (in Chapter 3), before a series of chapters explore global governance issues, including different types of actors, and the politics of global health (Chapters 4–7). Finally, Chapters 8–14 explore different areas where globalization and health intersect.

References

Barber, B. (1992) Jihad vs McWorld, *Atlantic Monthly*, 269 (3): 53–65.

Baylis, J., Smith, S. and Owens, P. (2008) *The Globalisation of World Politics*. Oxford: Oxford University Press.

Beck, U. (1999) *What is Globalization?* Cambridge: Polity Press.

Bozorgmehr, K. (2010) Rethinking the 'global' in global health: a dialectic approach, *Globalization and Health*, 6: 19.

Frenk, J. and Moon, S. (2013) Governance challenges in global health, *New England Journal of Medicine*, 368: 936–42.

Friedman, T. (1999) *The Lexus and the Olive Tree*. New York: HarperCollins.

Giddens, A. (1990) *The Consequences of Modernity*. Stanford, CA: Stanford University Press.

Harvey, D. (1989) *The Condition of Postmodernity*. Oxford: Blackwell.

Held, D. and McGrew, A. (2000) *The Global Transformations Reader*. London: Polity Press.

Held, D., McGrew, A., Goldblatt, D. and Perraton, J. (1999) *Global Transformations, Politics, Economics and Culture*. Stanford, CA: Stanford University Press.

Jenkins, R. (2004) Globalisation, production, employment and poverty: debates and evidence, *Journal of Development Studies*, 16: 1–12.

Khor, M. (1995) Globalization and the need for coordinated southern policy response, *Cooperation South, Special Issue*, pp. 15–18. New York: UNDP.

Koplan, J.P., Bond, T.C., Merson, M.H., Reddy, K.S., Rodriguez, M.H., Sewankambo, N.K. et al. (2009) Towards a common definition of global health, *Lancet*, 373 (9679): 1993–5.

Kruk, M. (2012) Globalisation and global health governance: implications for public health, *Global Public Health*, 7 (suppl. 1): S54–S62.

OECD (2008) Policy instruments to limit negative environmental impacts from increased international transport. Paper presented to the Global Forum on Transport and Environment in a Globalising World, 10–12 November 2008, Guadalajara, Mexico.

OECD (2012) *Trends in the Transport Sector 2012*. Paris: OECD.

Robertson, R. (1992) *Globalization: Social Theory and Global Culture*. London: Sage.

Scholte, J.A. (2000) *Globalization: A Critical Introduction*. London: Macmillan.

UNCTAD (2013) *Review of Maritime Transport 2013*. New York: United Nations Conference on Trade and Development.

UNDP (1999) *Human Development Report 1999*. New York: United Nations Development Programme.

2 Globalization, social change, and health

Andy Guise

Overview

Globalization is a process that influences all areas of our lives. Analysis of globalization often focuses on economic and political changes: the emergence of a global market economy, the expanding power of international financial institutions or multinational corporations, and the prominent role of specific countries within this economic integration. Globalization also has social impacts. If economics focuses on exchange of resources, politics on the governance of our societies, then sociological analysis refers to human life, groups, and societies (Giddens 2006). This chapter adopts a sociological perspective and explores how globalization is changing important aspects of our social lives, linked to political and economic changes, with significant implications for health, both good and bad.

Learning objectives

After working through this chapter, you will be able to:

- identify social changes linked to globalization and explore key concepts to help understand these
- understand the varying impacts these social changes have on health
- explore a specific case study of the health harms of illegal drugs and the impacts of globalization on gender

Key terms

Globalization: Increasing interconnections and relationships over space and time.

Global village: The idea that globalization is compressing space and time, creating shared experience.

Social determinants of health: The conditions in which people are born, grow, live, work, and age.

Analysing social change and health

Globalization is often understood as a process of increasing interconnections and relationships over space and time. While this is seen primarily to mean the emergence of a global marketplace and greater integration into a world economy (e.g. Labonte and

Schrecker 2009), it is also fundamentally about connections between people, and how we organize our societies and relate to each other. A powerful idea of social change resulting from globalization is that of the formation of a 'global village'. This is the idea that people are coming together, sharing values and beliefs, and forming a common humanity. This is an intuitive idea, capturing many people's experiences of feeling closer to others around the world. However, a range of social changes are linked with, and driven by, globalization. In this chapter, we will look across social life – where we live, our relationships with people, where we work, our norms and values – and explore changes in culture, identity, migration, urbanization, activism, citizenship, gender norms, and community relationships. The forces of globalization – increasing interconnections linked with global economic integration – are not the only factors involved in these social changes, but they are in differing ways catalyzing or intensifying them.

Changes in the social contexts in which we live have major impacts on our health. Our health is shaped by hereditary factors, which can, for example, increase our propensity for certain diseases. But health is also shaped by 'the conditions in which people are born, grow, live, work and age' (WHO 2008); we call these conditions the social determinants of health. Figure 2.1 summarizes the structures within which we live and which shape our health. Our focus in this chapter is the immediate social conditions in which people live, and which shape an individual's health. These social conditions mediate the overall political and economic structures of our societies: political and economic integration linked with globalization is felt, and changed, according to the specific conditions of where we live, where we work and who we are surrounded by.

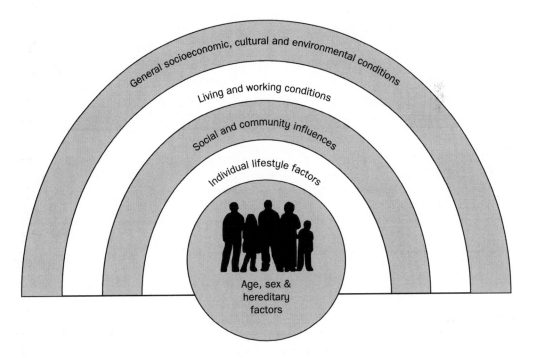

Figure 2.1 The determinants of health

Source: Dahlgren and Whitehead (1992)

Societies are complex phenomena, made up of hundreds, thousands or millions of people, and at a global scale, billions of people. Therefore, it is inevitable that the impact of globalization is complex. This complexity has an important meaning: simple conclusions of whether social change linked to globalization is good for health or not are misleading. The complexity of these processes leads to varied outcomes and inequalities. Globalization is creating enormous wealth and leading to increased differences in material wealth and opportunity, and linked differences in health. The WHO Commission on the Social Determinants of Health (2008) concluded that 'the social determinants of health are mostly responsible for health inequities – the unfair and avoidable differences in health status seen within and between countries'. This chapter approaches understanding the impact on health from the perspective that global economic and political integration has repercussions at the level of the home, the street, the workplace – where people live their lives. To understand the differential impact, we need to explore these in detail. A key theme across the chapter is how new social forms created through globalization create new spaces and opportunities in which some people's capacity to seek and have good health is improved, while for others it stays the same or deteriorates.

🖉 **Activity 2.1**

The WHO Commission for the Social Determinants of Health produced a report exploring how the daily conditions of life influence health and can be linked to health inequities. Globalization was a key theme in the report. Establishing causal relationships between globalization and health outcomes is difficult. Reflect on this challenge and from the report identify some forms and sources of evidence used. You can download the report from: http://www.who.int/social_determinants/thecommission/finalreport/en/.

Feedback

Just as the outcomes and impact of globalization are complex and varied, so too are the causes. Relating poor health outcomes to actions of single institutions, individuals, policies or processes is problematic. Social changes linked to globalization are long-term historical processes, making a focus on single causes and motivations simplistic. As such, there is a core methodological challenge in understanding how globalization impacts on health. A shift to increased integration into the global economy may impact health in a number of indirect ways that are challenging to catalogue. For example, some people may become poorer if they lose their job as a factory moves to another country, making health care less affordable. The complex causal relationships between social changes resulting from globalization and their impact on health have led to a lack of quality evidence. As the WHO Commission set out, it is impossible to do controlled trials or experiments in relation to globalization (you can't randomize countries – for ethical and practical reasons – to different policies to observe the impact). However, data and evidence do exist to allow us to build an understanding of individual relationships. The impact of environmental factors on childhood development is an example of this – carefully combining different data sources allows us to build insight into the health impact of globalization.

Key dimensions and concepts of social change

In the remainder of this chapter, we will examine four domains of social life: norms and values, living conditions, interpersonal relationships, and working environments. For each of these areas we will discuss concepts and processes that allow us to identify and explore key changes effected by globalization and their impact on health. The precise changes and impacts linked with these processes vary with space and time. The chapter ends with case studies of how globalization and social change are impacting on gender relations and the health harms associated with illicit drugs.

Norms and values

Many see globalization as leading to a global culture, with norms and values changing and evolving as societies become integrated into the global economy (Tomlinson 2007). Some view this process as a homogenizing force, with cultures becoming similar and less diverse: 'McDonaldization' is one label given to this process (Goodman 2007). The process of cultural change is linked to a dominant Western (often US) culture as evident in how iconic brands like McDonald's, Coca-Cola, and Marlboro are seen across the world (Tomlinson 2007).

Within this spread of global norms and adaptation there is a global trend towards a culture of consumerism (Goodman 2007). Primacy in this culture is focused on the wants and needs of the individual. Global consumerism is tied to multinational corporations and global brands. This process is linked to particular patterns of consumption of food, fashion, and ideas. The influence of Coca-Cola is a powerful example, how its global presence is part of not only an economic enterprise built around global value chains and infrastructure, but also the power of the cultural brand of Coca-Cola. These brands impact on our life-styles not by accident but through a deliberate effort to shape what people want. Lifestyles are generated via the creation of a brand through marketing. We can understand the power of advertising, as the ability to shape our perceptions and wants. This is not necessarily bad for health. Information about products is essential for us to make informed decisions. However, there are challenges to health when advertising promotes goods that are damaging to health, such as tobacco. Advertising is used to present tobacco as a product, and smoking as a lifestyle, that is part of a desirable western image. Figure 2.2 shows a tobacco advert from Indonesia drawing on images from the USA. This advert illustrates this process of drawing on global norms and values centring on western imagery.

The global obesity epidemic is a second example of how global cultural norms and global consumerism can negatively impact on health. Over a third of all adults are now considered obese or overweight, with the number of obese or overweight people in the developing world tripling between 1980 and 2008 (Keats and Wiggins 2014). This has a negative impact on health, for example, it can increase the risk of heart disease, diabetes, and some cancers. Obesity highlights the challenges resulting from global brands, corporations, and consumer lifestyles. We can see how a small number of organizations with significant cultural power are promoting particular lifestyles, which can be linked to the rise in consumption of high-energy and low-nutritional food. Comparisons have been made between the strategies employed by the 'big tobacco' and 'big food' companies to advertise their products, and companies promoting their products as having health benefits and publicly promoting doubt over the health risks posed by some products (Brownell and Warner 2009). This role of advertising in creating new norms around food consumption reflects a broader process of how the integration of the global economy is affecting diet, along with trade and production of food and investment in food processing and retail (Hawkes 2006).

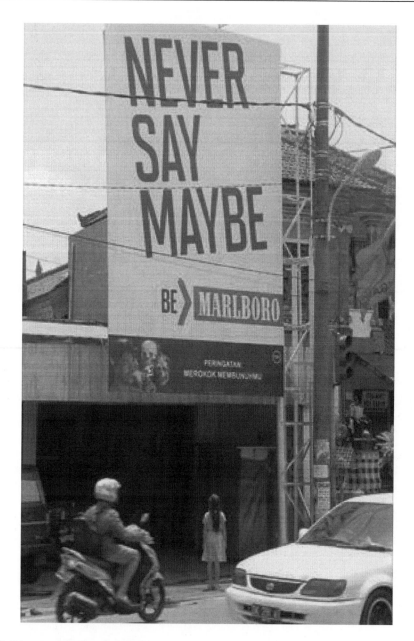

Figure 2.2 Tobacco advert from Indonesia

Source: Campaign for Tobacco-Free Kids, www.tobaccofreekids.org

---

Reflect on your own food consumption, and the extent to which the food you eat is both part of industrial processes and linked to global brands. Think about how much of what you eat is shaped by advertising and the lifestyles these adverts promote. How much of what you eat can be linked to norms and values that can be seen as global?

Feedback

In your considerations, you may be aware that you are eating products that are available in many different countries under the same brand, or products that have been produced in a different region of the world. Equally, you may make conscious choices about your food consumption such as buying things classified as 'organic' food, or you may choose to eat only locally produced food. These choices themselves may be the result of increased awareness or information enabled by greater communication and information flows resulting from globalization.

Living conditions

A central dimension of globalization shaping living conditions is migration. Estimates suggest there are 232 million migrants globally (IOM et al. 2013). Migration occurs for a range of reasons, including violence, conflict, and environmental degradation, but globalization is also a key factor (IOM et al. 2013). Travel and communication technologies increasingly allow people to move around the world to live in different places. This can be linked with improved work opportunities and access to health services, supporting good health. However, migration can also lead to marginalization within host countries and settings. Migrants can face increased barriers to accessing healthcare services, and also live in conditions that undermine good health. For example, migrants in to the European Union face a range of barriers to accessing health care, including fear and lack of awareness of their rights to care (Woodward et al. 2013).

Linked to migration, urbanization is another key social change driven by globalization. By 2010, more than half of the world's population lived in cities (WHO and UN-HABITAT 2010). Urbanization is a broader process resulting from rural–urban and cross-border migration, as well as natural growth of the populations in cities. Urbanization may also be a consequence of cities becoming a part of global chains of economic activity, particularly in terms of being a focus for foreign investment (Global Health Watch 2008) and the spread of technology and industry (WHO and UN-HABITAT 2010). Globalization is driving the formation of urban areas that have been labelled as 'superstar regions' (Perrons 2004). These are cities and urban areas that are the focus for global capitalism, and the political, corporate, and technical leadership linked with it. This concentration of power and functions in cities reflects a drive for coordination within a vast and complex global economy (Sassen 1991, in Perrons 2004).

Urban living creates opportunities and challenges for health. A negative side of urbanization is the increasing numbers of people living in informal settlements, or 'slums'. Cities like Johannesburg, Rio de Janeiro, Nairobi, Mumbai, and Jakarta are renowned for informal settlements characterized by poverty, situated in close proximity to the homes and offices of the wealthy, as in Figure 2.3. These cities have high inequality and spatial

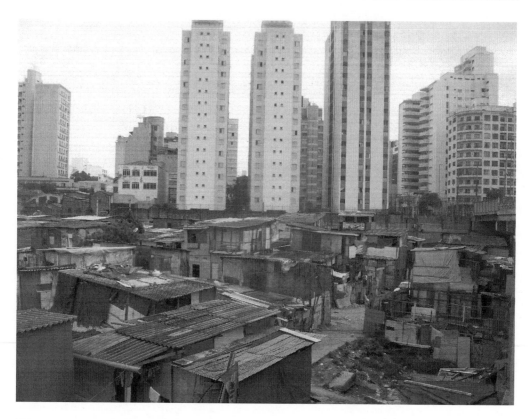

Figure 2.3 Social inequality: slums and skyscrapers, Brazil

exclusivity, increasingly in the form of gated communities and ghettos, with the poor marginalized in slum areas. Life in slums is frequently characterized by overcrowding, poor water and sanitation infrastructure, poor access to health care, as well as increased risk of violence and social conflict (WHO and UN-HABITAT 2010).

A concentration of populations brought by urbanization also creates positive opportunities for health. The principal reason is the increased potential for ease of access to services, with concentrations of people bringing economies of scale (UNFPA 2007). Providing care over large, remote areas is a logistical and financial challenge; major hospitals are after all found only in urban areas (Kebede-Francis 2011). Additional benefits to health come from the likelihood of improved access to sanitation and stable nutrition (Godfrey and Julien 2005). Despite the many downsides to health of urbanization, and slums in particular, considerable evidence suggests that health status is better on average for those in urban areas than rural areas (Godfrey and Julien 2005; WHO and UN-HABITAT 2010).

Interpersonal relationships

The idea of a global village suggests a level of connectivity and cohesion among people living in very different areas. There are indications of this cohesion forming, facilitated by information and communication technology (ICT). The telephone, the computer, and the Internet are key factors in this. Health-related activism in the form of social movements and non-governmental organizations (NGOs) such as the Treatment Action Campaign in South Africa and the World Social Forum can be seen as global organizations that transcend local or national boundaries. These movements bring together people from across the world to address both local and global health issues, whether in campaigning for particular local issues – for example, access to HIV treatment and care in South Africa – or in more global issues, like the right to health. An underlying process of this is the formation of global citizenship.

Citizenship refers to the membership of a group, and is usually framed in terms of the entitlements and obligations with reference to a nation-state and others living within the confines of that nation-state. A key question now is whether people are taking on global citizenship; the suggestion of this forming reflects how a globalized economy is weakening ties to specific territories (Falk 1999). One possible example of this global citizenship is the increased role for international NGOs and charities such as Médecins Sans Frontières (MSF) and the Red Cross. These organizations principally address health priorities in resource-poor settings, with funding and support by citizens from other areas. An emerging global consciousness is also reflected in the support for HIV treatment around the world. The fact that donors and key institutions like the Global Fund to fight AIDS, TB and Malaria are funding lifelong courses of therapy for HIV can be understood as a form of international solidarity (Ooms et al. 2010).

There are counter-arguments, however, to the formation of global citizenship. Some suggest this is just the case for elites (Falk 1999): an Internet connection and the time and resources to engage in global debates are perhaps the preserve of a relatively small number of people globally. Furthermore, international civil society is not necessarily benign; there are fascists and religious fundamentalists as much as women's movements and trades unions (Colás 1997), and so while protest groups can form to make progress on specific health issues, others can form to negate this, such as in groups forming across the Atlantic to question and undermine the science around the efficacy of MMR vaccinations (Goldacre 2009). The actions of globally functioning organizations can also be disruptive even if not intentionally so. There are profound concerns about the role of international NGOs in delivering health services in terms of whether they form part of an effective and sustainable health system. Critiques of international aid often cite how outside organizations prevent national governments from effectively coordinating and developing robust health systems (Vassall and Martínez Álvarez 2011).

✎ **Activity 2.3**

Do you think you live in a global village? In what ways are you connected to people locally, and also globally? What are the differences in these relationships?

Feedback

You may have considered where people in your neighbourhood are from, and that you work with people across different countries. Another form of global community that you may have considered is through online fora and social networking sites where you interact with people around a shared interest. Thus it encompasses both relationships virtually, as well as locally with the people in your community.

Working envivonment

A final area for consideration of social changes resulting from globalization is the conditions in which we work. These result from the economic integration associated with globalization and changing levels of wealth. Though employment and working conditions can provide financial security, social status, and personal development (WHO 2008), they can also be linked with material deprivation, acute psychosocial stress, income inequality, and social disintegration (Schrecker 2009).

The divisions of labour associated with the global economy are especially related to the formation of economic and, consequently, social inequalities. The global division of labour has resulted in low-tech labour-intensive production being relocated to developing countries owing to low wages and minimal protection for workers (Schrecker 2009), often highly damaging to health. Poor conditions can lead to exposure to toxins, long working hours which are physically and mentally exhausting, and expose workers to violence. Apple, the global producer of electronic goods, is one example of a multinational corporation outsourcing production that is linked with poor worker health (China Labour Watch 2013). These instances of negative impact on health through changing patterns of employment have to be balanced with data of how foreign ownership can be linked with better worker pay and conditions than domestically run businesses (Warren and Robertson 2011).

Box 2.1 Case study: Gender and work

Gender inequities exist in most if not all societies, principally leading to the marginalization of women and their increased vulnerability to ill health. Processes linked to globalization are challenging and changing existing gender norms. Market and trade liberalization has increased women's access to work, with potential benefits in terms of access to income and in turn autonomy over health and health care (Wamala and Kawachi 2007). There has been a shift in the balance across sectors, with women moving from work in agriculture to manufacturing and services. In developing countries, the share of service sector employment of women increased from 17 per cent in 1987 to 24 per cent in 2007 (World Bank 2011). However, these opportunities are often low paid and involve precarious working conditions, and can actually lead to a 'double burden' of work, with women taking on increased roles in the formal wage economy, while maintaining gender norms around domestic work and care (Wamala and Kawachi 2007). The increased migration of women to urban areas linked with their increasing role in services and manufacturing is similarly complex. While gender disparities in access to health and reproductive technologies in particular may be alleviated, inequities in vulnerability to ill health – such as HIV or violence – may be exacerbated (WHO and UN-HABITAT 2010).

✏ **Activity 2.4**

Consider the health risks and opportunities that might be faced by a young woman moving to an urban area in search of work. How would these differ from those faced by men?

Women may experience such benefits as better access to health services, reproductive health services, and greater autonomy resulting from wages. Risks may include exposure to unsafe working conditions, poor pay, a greater danger of violence, exploitation, and specific diseases. It may also extend to women facing a double burden of formal employment and domestic work, such as caring and housework traditionally associated with women. This is less likely to be a challenge for men moving to urban areas in search for work.

Box 2.2 Case study: A global risk environment for drugs

The health harms associated with illegal drugs show how social changes shaped by globalization are influencing health. The links between globalization and increased harm from illegal drugs have many dimensions. Perhaps most obviously, the illicit drug trade has benefited from globalization processes such as global transport technologies, reduced border controls, and the liberalization of financial markets (Singer 2008). More relevant for an analysis of social change is the argument that globalization exacerbates social inequality, creating an environment in which the poor turn to illegal drugs as a way to cope with and manage the 'injuries of globalization': stress, marginalization, and humiliation (Singer 2008). Alexander (2008) argues that the functioning of the global economy leads to greater individualism and social dislocation, which in turn fosters addiction as a means to cope. A loosening of traditional forms of control and support can be linked with increased drug use.

Rises in HIV rates in China as people inject heroin and share needles and syringes can be seen to result from the social changes created by the expanding market economy (Liu 2011). Greater mobility between rural and urban areas, and a breakdown in traditional ways of life, are leading men to migrate to urban centres in search of work. In these contexts, drugs are more widely available and men are away from the norms and social ties of rural life, making the use of heroin, for example, more likely. This is tied with emerging ideas and identities of how being a 'man' involves taking risks, and how taking drugs is seen as a symbol of fashion and affluence, and especially western ideals, which young men desire (Liu 2011).

This risk environment for drugs fostered by globalization is also evident in the Global North. In an ethnographic study of a Puerto Rican community in New York, Bourgois (2003) explores the lives and experiences of users and dealers of drugs, including crack cocaine and heroin. In exploring how individuals make decisions and act in ways that harm their health, Bourgois focuses on how the social environment structures and limits the decisions people can make. A history of migration to New York after eviction from rural areas in Puerto Rico by US agricultural companies is the basis for economic marginalization and low incomes, and social marginalization through racism. In this context, formal work in the mainstream economy is limited, leading people to the informal economy, crime, and involvement in drugs. The factors associated with the use of illegal drugs are numerous, but the social changes and structures linked with globalization are central to understanding why many people are using drugs and why communities can be damaged by them.

Summary

In this chapter, we have explored how globalization is leading to social changes, and in so doing impacting on health. The economic and political changes of globalization are being mediated through local-level social changes, whether it is the health of migrants, the alienation of city life or a rise in drug use. The ideas and concepts introduced in this chapter can be useful in understanding the detail of these changes, and in explaining why there are both winners and losers from globalization.

References

Alexander, B. (2008) *The Globalization of Addiction: A Study in Poverty of the Spirit*. Oxford: Oxford University Press.

Bourgois, P. (2003) *In Search of Respect: Selling Crack in El Barrio*. Cambridge: Cambridge University Press.

Brownell, K. and Warner, K. (2009) The perils of ignoring history: big tobacco played dirty and millions died. How similar is big food?, *Milbank Quarterly*, 87 (1): 259–94.

China Labour Watch (2013) *Beyond Foxconn: Deplorable Working Conditions Characterize Apple's Entire Supply Chain* [http://chinalaborwatch.org/pro/proshow-176.html]

Colás, A. (1997) The promises of international civil society, *Global Society*, 11 (3): 261–77.

Giddens, A. (2006) *Sociology* (5th edn). Cambridge: Polity Press.

Global Health Watch (GHW) (2008) *Global Health Watch 2: An Alternative World Health Report*. London: Zed Books.

Godfrey, R. and Julien, M. (2005) Urbanisation and health, *Clinical Medicine*, 5: 137–41.

Goldacre, B. (2009) *Bad Science*. London: Harper Perennial.

Goodman, D. (2007) Globalisation and consumer culture, in G. Ritzer (ed.) *The Blackwell Companion to Globalisation*, pp. 330–51. Oxford: Blackwell.

Falk, R. (1999) *Predatory Globalization: A Critique*. Cambridge: Polity Press.

Hawkes, C. (2006) Uneven dietary development: linking the policies and processes of globalization with the nutrition transition, obesity and diet-related chronic diseases, *Globalization and Health*, 2: 4 (DOI: 10.1186/1744-8603-2-4).

IOM, WHO and UNHCR (2013) *International Migration, Health and Human Rights*. Geneva: International Organisation for Migration, World Health Organization and United Nations Office of the High Commissioner for Human Rights.

Keats, S. and Wiggins, S. (2014) *Future Diets: Implications for Agriculture and Food Prices*. London: Overseas Development Institute.

Kebede-Francis, E. (2011) *Global Health Disparities*. Sudbury, MA: Jones & Bartlett Learning.

Labonte, R. and Schrecker, T. (2009) Introduction, in R. Labonte, T. Schrecker, C. Packer and V. Runnels (eds) *Globalisation and Health: Pathways, Evidence and Policy*. London: Routledge.

Liu, S. (2011) *Passage to Manhood: Youth Migration, Heroin and AIDS in Southwest China*. Stanford, CA: Stanford University Press.

Ooms, G., Hill, P., Hammonds, R., Van Leemput, L., Assefa, Y., Miti, K. et al. (2010) Applying the principles of AIDS 'exceptionality' to global health: challenges for global health governance, *Global Health Governance*, 4 (1): 1–9.

Perrons, D. (2004) *Globalisation and Social Change: People and Places in a Divided World*. London: Routledge.

Sassen, S. (1991) *The Global City*. Princeton, NJ: Princeton University Press.

Schrecker, T. (2009) Labour markets, equity and social determinants of health, in R. Labonte, T. Schrecker, C. Packer and V. Runnels (eds) *Globalisation and Health: Pathways, Evidence and Policy*, pp. 81–104. London: Routledge.

Singer, M. (2008) *Drugging the Poor: Legal and Illegal Drugs and Social Inequality*. Long Grove, IL: Waveland Press.

Tomlinson, J. (2007) Cultural globalization, in G. Ritzer (ed.) *The Blackwell Companion to Globalisation*, pp. 352–66. Oxford: Blackwell.

UNFPA (2007) *State of World Population 2007: Unleashing the Potential of Urban Growth*. New York: United Nations Population Fund.

Vassall, A. and Martínez Álvarez, M. (2011) The health system and external financing, in R. Smith and K. Hanson (eds) *Health Systems in Low and Middle Income Countries: An Economic and Policy Perspective*, pp. 193–218. Oxford: Oxford University Press.

Wamala, S. and Kawachi, I. (2007) Globalisation and women's health, in I. Kawachi and S. Wamala (eds) *Globalisation and Health*, pp. 171–84. Oxford: Oxford University Press.

Warren, C. and Robertson, R. (2011) Globalization, ages, and working conditions: a case study of Cambodian garment factories. CGD Working Paper 257. Washington, DC: Center for Global Development.

WHO (2008) *Closing the Gap in a Generation: Health Equity through Action on the Social Determinants of Health*. Geneva: World Health Organization.

WHO and UN-HABITAT (2010) *Hidden Cities: Unmasking and Overcoming Health Inequities in Urban Settings*. Geneva: World Health Organization.

Woodward, A., Howard, N. and Wolffers, I. (2013) Health and access to care for undocumented migrants living in the European Union: a scoping review, *Health Policy and Planning* (DOI: 10.1093/heapol/czt061).

World Bank (2011) Globalization's impact on gender equality: what's happened and what's needed, in *World Development Report 2012: Gender Equality*, pp. 254–78. Washington, DC: World Bank.

3 Introduction to the global economy

Kelley Lee

Overview

In this chapter, you will be introduced to economic globalization defined in terms of the changes taking place to world trade and finance. You will learn about two groupings of leading economies – the Group of Eight (G8) and Group of Twenty (G20) countries – and four institutional actors – the World Bank, the International Monetary Fund (IMF), the Organization for Economic Cooperation and Development (OECD), and the World Economic Forum (WEF), who are key to the governance of the world economy. A fifth, the World Trade Organization (WTO), will be discussed in Chapter 8, which focuses on the health impact of trade. Finally, the ongoing debate over whether economic globalization is good or bad for health is reviewed in relation to available evidence on economic growth, poverty and equity.

Learning objectives

After working through this chapter, you will be able to:

* define three types of economic globalization, and describe the shift from an international to a global economy
* understand the role of the G8, the G20, the World Bank, the IMF, the OECD, and the World Economic Forum in governing economic globalization
* describe the key debates on the positive and negative health effects of economic globalization

Key terms

Economic globalization: The process by which flows of goods and services, capital, labour or other means of production and exchange cross, and increasingly circumvent, national borders.

Global economy: An economy where production, exchange, and consumption are not linked to territorial distances but transcend national borders (trans-border).

International economy: An economy where production, exchange, and consumption take place across national borders between entities located in two or more countries (cross-border).

Three types of economic globalization

Before discussing the three types of globalization, we need to begin by distinguishing between two main components of economic globalization – trade and finance. Trade concerns the way in which goods and services are produced and exchanged between different countries. The globalization of trade means that there has been a *quantitative* increase in goods and services flowing between countries, as well as a *qualitative* change in the way they are produced. The globalization of finance refers to the increased quantity of currency trading, banking (savings and credit), and investment across countries, together with a qualitative change in how financial transactions are carried out. In other words, what we are seeing in trade and finance is both a greater intensity and reach of flows occurring across national borders and a greater number of countries and corporations involved in these flows.

Scholte (2000) identifies three types of economic globalization taking place (Table 3.1). Distinguishing among them helps to clarify frequent debates about whether globalization is occurring or not, the extent to which it is happening, and its time-frame.

The crossing of borders is what most people commonly refer to as economic globalization. This occurs when the production of a good or service takes place in Country A, and is then exported to consumers in Country B, Country C, and so on. For example, a South African factory may produce medical equipment in Cape Town. It might then export this equipment to hospitals in other countries on the African continent and beyond. This type of cross-border trade can be termed *internationalization.*

Trade between people across vast distances has taken place throughout human history (e.g. the Silk Route from the second millennium BC). When the modern system of states was formed in the seventeenth century, trade relations across societies became more complex. Trade boomed over the next two centuries as goods and services, capital, and even labour (e.g. slavery) were exchanged worldwide as part of the Industrial Revolution. Indeed, some writers argue that levels of cross-border trade (relative to total gross national product) actually rivalled the levels of trade we see today. People moved about without passports, trade flourished across distant continents, and the world economy grew rapidly. In this sense, it is sometimes argued that economic globalization, in the form of cross-border trade, is not really new.

The other two types of economic globalization described in Table 3.1, however, suggest that something more distinct has been happening from the mid to late twentieth century. The opening of borders, or trade *liberalization*, has accelerated rapidly since 1945. In the years leading up to the Second World War, many countries adopted policies that protected domestic industries and inhibited international trade in an effort to stimulate their own

Table 3.1 Three types of economic globalization

Crossing of borders (internationalization)	Increased cross-border movements between countries of people, goods, money, investments, messages, and ideas
Opening of borders (liberalization)	Progressive removal of border controls
Transcendence of borders (globalization)	Patterns of production, exchange, and consumption become increasingly delinked from geography of distances and borders

Source: Scholte (2000).

national economies. However, this worsened an already depressed world economy and, it has been argued, even contributed to the outbreak of war. The 44 Allied countries came together at Bretton Woods in the USA in 1944 (formally the United Nations Monetary and Financial Conference) to prevent a recurrence of such policies, and reached agreement to create three institutions: the World Bank, the IMF, and the General Agreement on Tariffs and Trade (GATT). The global health implications of trade liberalization will be covered later. Suffice to say here that trade liberalization policies promoted since the Second World War have led to the progressive removal of tariffs and other regulatory controls, thus encouraging international trade to flourish within the world economy.

The third type of economic globalization concerns the transcendence of borders, what Scholte (2000) defines more strictly as *globalization*. This term describes how certain flows of trade and finance have come to circumvent, and even ignore, territorial space or physical geography to the point of taking on a new economic logic. This transcendence of national borders by which the world as a whole becomes the scale of operation has been described by a number of writers. For example, in his book *Global Squeeze*, Longworth (1998) describes a Caterpillar plant in Toronto, Canada, that does not manufacture heavy machinery but rather assembles winches from Brazil, engines from Japan, axles from Belgium, and transmissions from the USA. The final product is then exported to markets worldwide. Similarly, the discovery in 2013 of horse meat in the human food chain across many European countries drew attention to the way that meat products have come to be manufactured, using basic foodstuffs and ingredients sourced from multiple countries, and sold in different markets around the world. As *Bloomberg News* (Editors 2013) reports: 'What's different today is that the food industry has become so sophisticated and supply chains so complex and global that it's much harder to monitor what goes into a product.'

As well as goods and services, economic globalization means the trans-border flow of finance. Indeed, financial markets have evolved to support globalized economic transactions. Perhaps the most significant event facilitating the emergence of a global financial system has been the so-called 'big bang' of the late 1980s, which was, in fact, a series of policies adopted to liberalize and deregulate the financial sector. It was a key event in the emerging global economy because it enabled currencies, credit, investments, and other financial assets to flow across the world with less attention to geography. Between 2004 and 2013, cross-border foreign exchange transactions increased from about US$1.5 trillion to US$5.3 trillion average daily turnover (BIS 2013). Liberalization of financial flows by governments around the world has further encouraged such flows of capital, outpacing growth in world trade during the same period.

A good illustration of financial globalization is the Royal Bank of Scotland Group (also known as RBS Group), a British banking and insurance holding company based in Edinburgh. Operating throughout Europe, North America, and Asia, the group offers personal and business banking, private banking, insurance, and corporate finance. RBS was briefly the largest bank in the world, prior to the global financial crisis in 2008, although its share price has fallen sharply since due to continued uncertainty in the world's financial markets. Thousands of individuals choose to invest in specialized funds under its management. Many funds are global in reach, with fund managers buying shares in different companies across many economic sectors based around the world. There is a lot of buying and selling of shares as the bank tries to earn the best return for its individual and institutional clients from these different companies. Multiply these transactions billions of times over and we gain a sense of the change that has happened to investment activity worldwide. Today, money handed to a financial advisor is, in short, destined to join a global investment system that truly transcends borders.

Table 3.2 Royal Bank of Scotland Emerging Markets Equity Fund

Company	Sector	Country	% of assets
Samsung Electronics	Information technology	South Korea	4.5
Taiwan Semiconductor Manufacturing	Information technology	Taiwan	3.9
Housing Development Financing Corp Ltd.	Property	India	3.6
SABMiller Plc	Food and drink	UK	3.1
China Mobile Ltd.	Telecommunications	China	3.0
Sberbank of Russia Ltd.	Financial	Russia	2.9
PetroChina Company Ltd.	Energy	China	2.8
Embotelladora Andina SA	Food and drink	Chile	2.7
Public Bank Bhd	Financial	Malaysia	2.7
AIA Group Ltd.	Financial	China	2.5

Source: RBS Global Asset Management, *Emerging Markets Equity Fund*. Available at: http://fundinfo.rbcgam.com/ mutual-funds/rbc-funds/fund-pages/rbf499.fs

One of the investment funds that RBS offers is its Emerging Markets Equity Fund whose investment objective is '[t]o provide long-term capital growth. The fund invests primarily in equity securities of companies located or active in emerging markets.' Its top ten holdings (31.2 per cent of holdings) in December 2013 were as shown in Table 3.2. This indicates the truly global nature of a typical bank.

There remains much debate about the timing of the global economy's emergence, and the extent to which it is happening across different sectors. Available evidence suggests that economic globalization is occurring more readily in certain health-related sectors such as pharmaceuticals, medical technologies, food and beverages, financial services, and tobacco and alcohol. In other sectors, such as health care, it is happening to a more limited degree, although the growth of medical tourism suggests a growing international trade in health care services. In the early twenty-first century, therefore, it may be more accurate to describe the world economy as 'globalizing' rather than 'globalized'. Some sectors lend themselves to being 'globalized' because they do not require one geographical base, or may benefit from economies of scale or production across different geographical locations. Others may remain heavily regulated by national authorities, for social or other reasons, and will thus remain relatively attached to particular geographical territories.

✐ **Activity 3.1**

Purchase a print copy of a national newspaper in your country or a major international newspaper such as the *International Herald Tribune, New York Times* or *Le Monde*. Ensure that the newspaper has a business section.

1 Scan the business section and see what proportion of the stories is concerned with locally based versus globally operating companies.
2 Can you identify an example of an 'internationalized' company that has its main operations in one country but exports its goods and/or services to other coun-

tries? Confirm your assessment by looking on the company's website. Look out for a company that is important to health, for example, a company trading in pharmaceuticals, alcohol or food.

3 Can you identify an example of a 'globalized' company that organizes different parts of its operations in different geographical locations? What parts of the production chain are carried out where? Where does the company source and process raw materials? Where are the company's major markets for its product(s)? Confirm your assessment by looking on the company's website.

Feedback

You should observe that internationalized companies produce goods and/or services in one country and export them to other countries. They may also set up facilities to produce goods and/or services in other countries, which may be used to supply the domestic market or to export to other countries. You should then distinguish such operations from global companies that locate different parts of the production chain in different locales. The goods and/or services produced would then supply various markets worldwide. These types of companies illustrate an increasingly integrated global economy.

Who are the big players in the global economy?

Strong evidence of an emerging global economy is the growth in companies that operate in more than one country. Definition is important here. The terms 'multinational corporation' and 'transnational corporation' are often used interchangeably, or can be defined differently in different professions, which makes it difficult to analyse trends. But when talking about economic globalization, it is useful to distinguish between the two.

A *multinational* corporation (MNC), company or enterprise can be loosely defined as one which is registered, or has registered operations, in more than one country. It is generally headquartered in one 'home' country, and operates subsidiaries in 'host' countries. Subsidiaries may replicate the parent company's operations but primary decision-making power remains at headquarters. It was estimated that MNCs increased from around 3000 in 1990 (Gabel and Bruner 2003) to over 65,000 (including 850,000 subsidiaries) by 2013 (Cullen and Praveen Parboteeah 2013).

A *transnational* corporation (TNC) is qualitatively different because it does not identify itself with a single national home. Instead, it operates a more decentralized pattern of production and exchange, with decision-making taken by senior executives of different nationalities based on a business strategy from a global perspective. Definitional imprecision makes it difficult to provide an accurate estimate of numbers of TNCs over time worldwide. Many companies are also transitioning, from an international to global business strategy. Evidence suggests a rapid growth of TNCs in selected sectors as true economic globalization occurs.

Importantly, a globalizing world economy means not only that there are more MNCs and TNCs, but also that these companies are becoming more economically powerful. Today, some sectors have become dominated by a few very large companies, many commanding resources comparable to entire countries. Figure 3.1 shows that General Electric was the largest company in the world in 2011 with US$725 billion in assets (over US$500 billion in foreign assets).

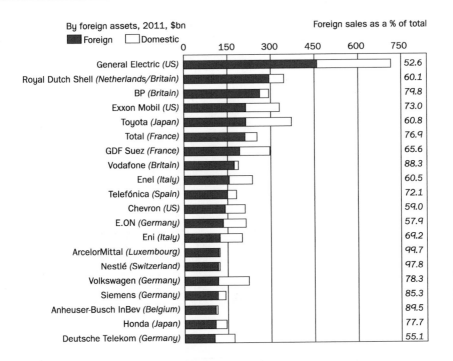

Figure 3.1 The world's largest transnational companies, 2011

Source: The Economist, 10 July 2012 [http://www.economist.com/blogs/graphicdetail/2012/07/focus-1]

Table 3.3 Top ten companies by profits earned, 2012

Company	Profits (US$ million)	% change in profits since 2000
Exxon Mobil	44,880.0	153
Apple	41,733.0	6844
GazProm	38,086.2	1665
Industrial & Commercial Bank of China	37,806.5	5895
China Construction Bank	30,618.2	3262
Volkswagen	27,909.1	1372
Royal Dutch Shell	26,592.0	109
Chevron	26,179.0	405
Agricultural Bank of China	22,996.9	53,506
Bank of China	22,099.5	3894

Source: Compiled from CNN Money (2012) *Fortune Global 500: 2012*. Retrieved from: http://money.cnn.com/magazines/fortune/global500/2012/full_list/

By total revenues, Royal Dutch Shell is the world's largest TNC with US$470 billion in total revenues (including US$283 billion in foreign revenues), followed by Exxon Mobil (US$432 billion in total revenues) and Walmart Stores (US$422 billion) (UNCTAD 2012). Ranked by profit (Table 3.3), Exxon Mobil led the world economy with US$44.9 billion (compared with US$17.7 billion in 2000), followed by Apple (US$41.7 billion) and GazProm (US$38 billion) in 2012 (*Fortune Global 500*, 8 July 2013). The size of these companies is now comparable to the gross domestic products of entire countries such as Lebanon and Lithuania (US$42 billion) and Ghana (US$40 billion) in 2012.

Key institutions governing economic globalization

How did we get to where we are today? Has this happened 'naturally', as neoliberal economic theorists would argue, by allowing market forces to find efficiencies through greater economies of scale and optimal returns within and across countries? Can we see the growth of these ever-larger corporations, operating across geographical boundaries, as the result of an economic 'survival of the fittest' within a more competitive world market? Does this greater efficiency mean that this is an economic trend generating greater wealth and prosperity, and thus should be encouraged? Some writers argue that the 'invisible hand' of the market is rationalizing economies worldwide. Economic globalization, in this sense, is seen as the triumph of capitalism writ large, a progressive force driven by basic economic principles. And like boats rising with an incoming tide, it is argued that increased wealth worldwide will ultimately benefit everyone (Lal 2006).

Many critics of existing forms of economic globalization, however, dispute this explanation, arguing that the increased domination of the world economy by larger and fewer companies is the result of deliberate policy decisions, embedded within existing institutional structures and processes, to benefit certain interests over others. This perspective holds that there is nothing rational or inevitable about how economic globalization has emerged and spread. Instead, it has been driven by vested interests and ideological principles, which in turn have defined the nature and direction of economic globalization. The result has been a particular, and many argue unjust, distribution of the benefits and costs generated by globalization (Falk 1999).

It is beyond the scope of this book to describe in detail all the relevant institutions concerned with the governance of economic globalization. However, a basic understanding of the World Bank, the IMF, and the World Economic Forum provides an important starting point for understanding how the world economy has come to be structured as it is today. The role of the World Trade Organization (WTO) in relation to trade and health is addressed in Chapter 8.

While the roots of the world economy can be traced back centuries, events leading up to and after the Second World War institutionalized the main principles and practices that define economic globalization today. A key factor contributing to the outbreak of war in 1939 was the world economic crisis. Beginning with the crash of stock markets known as Black Thursday (29 October 1929), followed by the worst economic depression in world history, country after country tried to boost their domestic economies by adopting protectionist trade policies such as higher tariffs on imports, import quotas, and foreign exchange controls. These policies, often referred to as 'tit for tat' or 'beggar thy neighbour' policies, in fact worsened the economic climate across the world, contributing further to a worldwide economic downturn.

The harsh lessons from these events, which saw industrial production across the world drop by up to 47 per cent, led the leaders of the Allied countries to create a new economic order that would ensure stability, trade, and economic growth. A conference was held in Bretton Woods, New Hampshire, in 1944 to create the institutions that would govern this new world economy.

World Bank

The World Bank was created initially to support the rebuilding of economies devastated during the Second World War. Financed and governed by its member states, its initial role was defined as providing loans to countries for basic infrastructure such as dams, roads, and power plants. Backed by major governments as guarantors, the Bank borrowed funds on the commercial markets with interest, and then re-loaned these funds to applicant countries at a slightly higher interest rate to ensure a small return. There was a need for the World Bank, as the lender of last resort, because it could provide loans to countries with limited access to commercial financing and at competitive rates.

The World Bank actually consists of a group of five institutions with the following functions:

1 to provide 'soft' loans at low or no interest to the poorest countries (International Development Association);
2 to support private sector investment in World Bank-approved projects (International Finance Corporation);
3 to provide risk insurance to foreign companies seeking to invest in member states (Multilateral Insurance Guarantee Agency);
4 to provide facilities for conciliation and arbitration of international investment disputes involving member states (International Centre for Settlement of Investment Disputes);
5 to promote development through loans, guarantees, risk management products, and analytical and advisory services (International Bank for Reconstruction and Development).

The latter is the branch most commonly referred to as the 'World Bank' and, as such, has been subject to the greatest scrutiny. For health development purposes, the International Development Association is also important because it provides medium- to long-term loans at very low interest to the poorest countries. More recently, amid a growing number of bilateral investment treaties (BITs), and the increased importance of large companies in the global economy, the International Centre for Settlement of Investment Disputes has become increasingly important for settling claims brought by companies against governments.

Formally, the World Bank (like the IMF) is a specialized agency of the UN system, but historically it has acted independently. This is reflected in its membership and decision-making processes. The World Bank, like other UN specialized agencies, consists of member states who formally take part in decision-making. But, unlike other UN specialized agencies which are ruled by the 'one state, one vote' principle, World Bank voting rights are based on a member state's financial contribution. Under this rule, in 2013 high-income countries held around 61 per cent of votes, middle-income countries 35 per cent, and low-income countries 4.46 per cent. The Bank is headed by a Board of Governors consisting of a Governor and alternate Governor appointed by each of the 188 member states. The country's minister of finance, governor of its central bank or a senior official of similar rank usually holds this office. Beneath this, and where the real power lies, is the Board of Directors, comprised of Executive Directors drawn from a select group of 25 member states and the elected World Bank President, that is tasked with making key decisions. The Bank operates under the leadership and direction of the President, who is customarily an American citizen, and organizational units responsible for regions, sectors, and general management. Three Managing Directors also oversee operations, working with over 9000 multidisciplinary staff from more than 168 countries based at headquarters in Washington, DC, and around 100 country offices worldwide. Staff are organized by Vice Presidential Units (VPUs) including six regional vice presidencies and four thematically based networks. Health development experts are based in both the regional units and networks (see Figure 3.2).

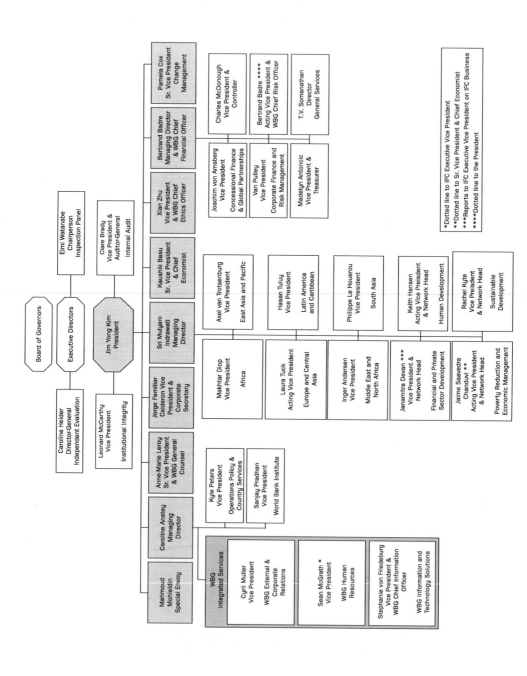

Figure 3.2 Organizational chart of the World Bank, effective 1 July 2013

Source: World Bank (2013) [http://siteresources.worldbank.org/EXTABOUTUS/Resources/bank.pdf]

The World Bank Group's importance to economic globalization stems from its capacity to provide financing to developing economies (around US$53 billion in 2012). While loans are ostensibly to promote growth and overcome poverty, as a lender of last resort the Bank has the power to set certain requirements of borrowing governments (known as policy conditionalities), deemed necessary to achieve these goals, before financing is issued.

Controversially, from the early 1980s, policy conditionality focused on making national economies 'leaner and meaner', under so-called structural adjustment programmes (SAPs), and to integrate them into the emerging global economy. It was held that if borrowing countries strengthened competition within private markets, supported trade liberalization, reduced public spending, and encouraged foreign direct investment, this would generate economic growth and thus bring benefits to all. Almost immediately, however, such policies were criticized for failing to take sufficient account of their wider social and environmental consequences. Evidence from a wide variety of contexts suggested adverse health effects:

- In Tanzania, a series of adjustment programmes adopted from 1981 were found to have contributed to increased maternal mortality, chronic malnutrition, and poverty (Lugella 1995).
- In China, the introduction of user fees for tuberculosis treatment resulted in some 1.5 million cases being left untreated, leading to an additional 10 million people becoming infected (Werner and Sanders 1997).
- In Costa Rica, a 35 per cent cut in health programmes under the SAP was followed by a dramatic increase in infectious disease rates and infant mortality (Peabody 1996).
- In South Africa, the introduction of water charges under the SAP is believed to have led to a serious outbreak of cholera in eastern KwaZulu-Natal in 2001 (Scrace 2006).

Despite wide-ranging criticism, the World Bank has remained one of the core institutional pillars of market-driven strategies to promote economic globalization. Cognisant of the concerns levied against it, there have been efforts to give greater attention to good governance, poverty reduction, sustainability, and social capital as important development goals. Nonetheless, debates remain about the nature of the loans it provides, the policy conditionalities attached, and the structure of decision-making that governs its activities.

International Monetary Fund

The International Monetary Fund (IMF) was created as an independent international organization to promote world economic stability and growth. Its mandate is:

- to promote international monetary cooperation through a permanent institution which provides the machinery for consultation and collaboration on international monetary problems;
- to facilitate the expansion and balanced growth of international trade, and to contribute thereby to the promotion and maintenance of high levels of employment and real income and to the development of the productive resources of all members as primary objectives of economic policy;
- to promote exchange stability, to maintain orderly exchange arrangements among members, and to avoid competitive exchange depreciation;

- to assist in the establishment of a multilateral system of payments in respect of current transactions between members and in the elimination of foreign exchange restrictions that hamper the growth of world trade;
- to give confidence to members by making the general resources of the IMF temporarily available to them under adequate safeguards, thus providing them with the opportunity to correct maladjustments in their balance of payments without resorting to measures destructive of national or international prosperity; and
- to shorten the duration and lessen the degree of disequilibrium in the international balances of payments of members.

Its main stated functions are:

- to maintain surveillance over members' economic policies;
- to finance temporary balance of payment needs;
- to mobilize external funding;
- to strengthen the international monetary system; and
- to increase the supply of global currency reserves.

In practice, the IMF is described as a cooperative of shareholders that provides capital largely through quota subscriptions. *Quota subscriptions* are a central component of the IMF's financial resources, assigned to each member state according to its relative position in the world economy. The quota determines a country's maximum financial commitment to the IMF, its voting power, and access to IMF financing via 'special drawing rights'[1] if needed. In return, the IMF provides member states with macroeconomic policy advice, financing in times of balance of payments need, and technical assistance and training to improve national economic management. These functions were generally supported by the international community given the clear need for an effective mechanism to solve short-term currency imbalances in national economies, a function increasingly important as economic globalization has spread.

Criticisms of the IMF, however, have been similar to those levied at the Bank, namely its governance structure and, relatedly, appropriateness of its policy conditionalities. The IMF is formally governed by a Board of Governors, the highest decision-making body of the organization, consisting of one Governor (usually a minister of finance or equivalent official) and an alternate Governor from each of the 185 member states. The main policy-making organ of the IMF, however, is the Executive Board (supported by a number of standing committees), which is responsible for the conduct of day-to-day business, including the approval of all IMF lending operations. The 24-member Executive Board is chaired by the Managing Director, customarily a European citizen and selected by the Executive Board. Like the World Bank, decision-making power (number of votes) is weighted according to a member state's economic status. The five countries with the largest quotas can appoint their own Executive Director, along with the two largest creditors. The remaining board members are elected by member states. The IMF employs around 2400 staff, around half of whom are economists.

The weighting of decision-making in the IMF in favour of the most economically powerful has been widely criticized. Of particular concern has been the organization's ability, like the World Bank, to make lines of credit 'conditional upon the achievement of economic stabilization and structural reform objectives' (IMF 2001). Like the Bank, the IMF has promoted neoliberal-based economic principles with varied effects at best. These principles, summarized as a set of policy ideas known as the Washington Consensus (because many of the institutions behind them are based in Washington, DC) are:

- fiscal discipline
- redirection of public expenditure
- tax reform
- financial liberalization
- single competitive exchange rates
- trade liberalization
- elimination of barriers to foreign direct investment
- privatization of state-owned enterprises
- deregulation of market entry and competition
- assurance of secure property rights.
  (Williamson 1990)

Focused on international trade and economic growth, critics argue that little attention has been paid to the social and environmental consequences of such strategies. Other concerns raised relate to the IMF's tendency to apply the same policy requirements to different country needs and contexts, its lack of accountability, and its lending to governments with poor human rights records. Further scrutiny and pressures to reform the IMF, as a key institutional player in managing economic globalization, have been prompted by its handling of financial crises including the global financial crisis from 2008.

Organization for Economic Cooperation and Development

The Organization for Economic Cooperation and Development (OECD) was created to 'promote polices that will improve the economic and social well-being of people around the world' (OECD n.d.). Initially established in 1948 as the Organization for European Economic Cooperation (OEEC), its original aim was to aid European recovery after the Second World War under the Marshall Plan. After Canada and the USA became members, joining eighteen European countries, the OECD was officially created on 30 September 1961 with its headquarters in Paris.

There are currently 34 member states of the OECD. Article 16 of the OECD's Convention states:

> The Council may decide to invite any Government prepared to assume the obligations of membership to accede to this Convention. Such decisions shall be unanimous, provided that for any particular case the Council may unanimously decide to permit abstention, in which case, notwithstanding the provisions of Article 6, the decision shall be applicable to all the Members. Accession shall take effect upon the deposit of an instrument of accession with the depositary Government.
>
> (OECD 1960)

It is not specified in the Convention how the accession process should take place; and it was not until 2007 that the OECD formalized a strategy for enlargement and an accession process, with Chile being the first new member country to follow the process (Carroll and Aynsley 2011). In 2010, Chile, Slovenia, Israel, and Estonia joined after almost three years of accession process. The perceived exclusivity of OECD membership, limited to high-income or major emerging economies, has been the subject of criticism.

The role of the OECD is to provide a forum where member states can collaborate and pursue potential solutions to shared problems, by sharing their economic experiences. Its specific functions are:

- to work with governments to understand what leads to economic, social, and environmental change;
- to measure productivity and global flows of trade and investment;
- to utilize and analyse collected data to produce future trend estimates; and
- to set a variety of international standards including issues such as tax, agriculture, and chemical safety.

The OECD consists of three main bodies: the Council, Committees, and the Secretariat (Figure 3.3). Decision-making is taken by the Council, based on consensus among representatives of its member states and the European Commission. Discussion of specific policy areas, such as health policy, occurs within approximately 250 committees and working groups. The administration of the OECD's work is undertaken by the Secretariat headed by the Secretary-General, who chairs the Council, Deputy Secretaries-General, and Directorates, and around 2500 Paris-based staff (primarily economists).

In relation to health policy, the OECD compiles a wide range of data from member states, presented in the annual *OECD Health Data* and *Health at a Glance* reports, including health status indicators, non-medical determinants of health, health care resources and utilization, pharmaceutical production and consumption (including generic drugs), long-term care resources and utilization, health expenditure, and demographic and economic references. Based on recognition of the importance of the health sector to economic development policy, OECD data and analysis have been perceived as increasingly important to policy-makers and analysts.

Council
Oversight and strategic direction

Representatives of member countries and of the European Commission; chaired by the Secretary-General; decisions taken by consensus

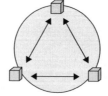

Committees
Discussion and implementation

Representatives of member countries and of countries with Observer status work with the OECD Secretariat on specific issues

Secretariat
Analysis and proposals

Secretary-General
Deputy Secretaries-General
Directorates

Figure 3.3 The structure of the OECD

Source: OECD [http://www.oecd.org/about/whodoeswhat/]

World Economic Forum

The World Economic Forum (WEF) describes itself as 'an independent international organization committed to improving the state of the world by engaging business, political, academic and other leaders of society to shape global, regional and industry agendas' (World Economic Forum n.d.). It seeks to provide a collaborative framework for the world's leaders to address global issues, engaging corporate members in particular in 'global

Table 3.4 Member organizations of the World Economic Forum by region, 2005

Region	No. of members	% of total
Europe	430	43
North America	262	26
Asia	131	13
Central/South America	75	7
Middle East	45	4
Africa	43	4
Australasia	22	2

Source: Compiled from data on the WEF website [www.weforum.org]

citizenship'. Boasting membership of over 1000 of the world's leading companies, usually 'with over $5 billion in turnover', it is difficult to dispute its status as 'the foremost global community of business, political, intellectual and other leaders of society'. The WEF holds a wide range of regional and international meetings, with the most well-known being its annual meeting in Davos, Switzerland, which brings together around 2000 'of the most knowledgeable, dynamic and influential people in the world' from more than 100 countries. In 2007, the foundation established the Annual Meeting of the New Champions (also called Summer Davos), held annually in China, convening 1500 Global Growth Companies, primarily from rapidly growing emerging countries such as China, India, Russia, Mexico, and Brazil, but also rapidly growing companies from developed countries. Health-related work includes the Global Health Initiative launched by the UN Secretary-General in 2002, to engage businesses in public–private partnerships to tackle HIV/AIDS, tuberculosis, and malaria. Since 2000, the WEF has also highlighted social entrepreneurship as a key element to advance societies and address social problems.

Criticisms of the WEF focus on its perceived elitist membership. A regional breakdown of its 1007 member organizations (Table 3.4) in 2005 reflects the concentration of the world's wealth in high-income countries. While much has been done since to ensure broader geographical representation in WEF events, largely in response to demands from major emerging economies, what remains reflected in WEF membership is a clear divide between the 'haves' and 'have nots' within the global economy.

As an alternative, since 2001 civil society organizations have held an annual World Social Forum that challenges this elite 'to listen to the needs and concerns of poorer communities and provides an opportunity for campaigners from across the globe to meet' (Christian Aid 2002). The forum is envisioned as

an open meeting place for reflective thinking, democratic debate of ideas, formulation of proposals, free exchange of experiences and interlinking for effective action, by groups and movements of civil society that are opposed to neoliberalism and the domination of the world by capital and any form of imperialism, and are committed to building a planetary society directed towards fruitful relationships among humans and those with the Earth.

(World Social Forum 2001)

The Occupy Movement, an international protest against social and economic inequality, has also sought to challenge the marked skewing of the world's wealth. Its slogan, 'We are the 99%' refers to the heavy concentration of wealth in one per cent of populations. This one per cent is what critics have described as 'Davos man', a transnational class of the political and economic elite, characterized by its control of political and economic power rather than its geographical location, and which has come to dominate economic globalization.

Activity 3.2

How does the WEF differ from the World Social Forum (WSF) in terms of purpose and participation? Compare the websites of the two organizations regarding their membership and ways they contribute.

Feedback

The stated purpose of the WEF (see above) contrasts with that of the WSF, which describes itself as 'an open meeting place for reflective thinking, democratic debate of ideas, formulation of proposals, free exchange of experiences and inter-linking for effective action, by groups and movements of civil society that are opposed to neo-liberalism and to domination of the world by capital and any form of imperialism, and are committed to building a society centred on the human person'. Participation in the WSF is by civil society organizations from all countries. However, participants are not called on to take decisions as a body, whether by vote or acclamation, on declarations or proposals for action that would commit all, or the majority, of them to it. Rather, it is open to a diversity of views, activities, and ways of engaging of the organizations and movements that decide to participate, as well as to the diversity of genders, ethnicities, cultures, generations, and physical capacities represented in the Forum.

Group of Eight and Group of Twenty countries

The Group of Eight (G8) plays a key role in global economic governance. Initially launched as the G5 (US, Germany, UK, France, and Japan) in 1974, following the 1971 collapse of the Bretton Woods system, the group expanded to become the G6 in 1975 (adding Italy), G7 in 1976 (adding Canada), and then the G8 in 1998 (adding Russia). The G8 is less structured than the World Bank or the OECD, for example; it is organized without a formal international agreement or secretariat, yet meets regularly to make decisions on key global economic matters (Hajnal 2007).

The stated roles of the G8 are 'deliberation, direction-giving, and decision-making as well as global governance and domestic political management functions' (Hajnal 2007: 32). At its annual summits, the leaders of the G8 countries have dealt with issues around macroeconomic management, international trade, and relations with developing countries. In more recent years, microeconomic issues, transnational issues encompassing the environment, crime, and drugs, and political-security issues such as arms control and human rights security have been given considerable attention on summit agendas (The G8 Research Group 2012).

The small number of member states allows the building of personal relationships and trust, hence the enabling of candid and freewheeling discussion on sensitive political issues. At the same time, the membership has been criticized as an exclusive club of the world's wealthiest governments whose deliberations have worldwide impacts. In an attempt to address concerns about representation, key developing countries (Brazil, China, India, Mexico, and South Africa) were invited to the 2005 G8 Summit in Gleneagles, Scotland, thus expanding the group to the so-called 'G8+5' (Smith 2011).

Expanding membership further, the Group of Twenty (G20) was created as an informal group consisting of 19 countries (the G8 and key regional powers) and the European Union, along with representatives from the World Bank and IMF. Formed in 1999, it was preceded by similar efforts to form a G22 in 1998 and a G33 in 1999 (Hajnal 2007; The G20 Research Group 2010). In addition to the G8 countries, Argentina, Australia, Brazil, China, India, Indonesia, Mexico, Saudi Arabia, South Africa, South Korea, and Turkey are G20 member countries. Reflecting the economic focus of the agenda, the G20 initially comprised finance ministries, rather than heads of state. The G20's main objective was to create a mechanism in which financial and economic policy issues would be discussed among key economies (Hajnal 2007). This was changed in 2008 when then US President George W. Bush called the leaders of the G20 countries together to organize the first G20 summit as a global response to the US financial crisis (OECD 1960; The G20 Research Group 2010). The G20 agenda has since shifted, from a heavy focus on economic issues to addressing the opportunities and challenges of globalization, global poverty, the UN Millennium Development Goals (MDG), employment, and demographic change (Hajnal 2007).

The issue of representation and legitimacy of the G8 has to a certain extent been addressed by the presence of the G20. The G20 represents all the world regions; and the member countries account for two-thirds of the world population and some 90 per cent of GDP globally (Hajnal 2007). Nevertheless, criticism remains around the lack of representation by the world's poorest peoples.

In summary, the World Bank, the IMF, the OECD and the WEF, alongside the G8 and the G20, are key pillars of contemporary economic globalization. The global financial crisis from 2008 has raised substantive concerns about the social, environmental, and indeed economic impacts of the 'boom' and 'bust' cycles created by free market-driven policies and the absence of effective global regulatory frameworks. The crisis has also renewed debates about the governance of these key institutions in terms of their accountability, transparency, and representation in decision-making processes. This is specifically the case with the rise in new global powers, such as Brazil, Russia, India, China, and South Africa, commonly referred to collectively as the BRICS countries. The incorporation of the BRICS countries expands the number of countries governing the global economy, but there remain concerns as to whether they are simply joining or replacing the existing elite, rather than ushering in a new world economic order. Institutional reform, and the achievement of good global economic governance more generally, remain a core challenge.

Is economic globalization good or bad for health?

The short answer is both. However, there remains great debate about economic globalization concerning its true impacts on people's lives, and in particular the capacity to improve the lives of the world's poor. This is a highly polarized debate and it lies at the heart of so-called anti-globalization demonstrations. The key dispute is whether the global economy, as currently structured and directed, is a positive or negative force for human development and environmental sustainability as exemplified by the following quotes:

> anyone who cares about the poor should favor the growth-enhancing policies of good rule of law, fiscal discipline, and openness to international trade.
>
> (Dollar and Kraay 2001)

> the new feature of market economics in present day capitalism . . . [is] turbo-capitalism . . . Whoever thinks that the stability of families and communities is important cannot at the same time speak in favour of deregulation and globalization of the economy.
>
> (Luttwak 1996, in Martin and Schumann 1997)

Supporters of current forms of economic globalization might be described as 'globalists'. Globalists support what can neatly be summarized as a set of policy ideas known as the Washington Consensus (described above). This set of ideas has, for example, underpinned structural adjustment programmes, responses to regional and global financial crises, and development aid since the early 1980s.

On the link between globalization and health, globalists would argue that:

- liberalization increases flows of trade and finance;
- trade increases growth, especially in poorer countries;
- growth increases incomes, especially for the poor, so eventually there is a convergence of wealth (i.e. the trickle-down effect);
- higher incomes mean more resources for governments to spend on health services; and
- higher incomes for the poor means better living conditions and hence improved health status.

These assumed causal links lead to the overall conclusion that globalization is good for health. Globalists argue that all countries need to integrate with the emerging global economy, and where some countries suffer adverse effects, it is because they have not embraced globalization sufficiently.

What evidence supports these policy prescriptions? The work of Dollar and colleagues (Dollar and Kraay 2001; Dollar et al. 2013) is seminal in this debate. They argue that countries that have embraced economic globalization over the past two decades have benefited most. Less globalized countries have suffered negative growth in GDP, while more globalized poor countries have enjoyed growth (over 5 per cent) higher even than high-income countries (Figure 3.4). Over the past forty years, they argue, more globalized countries have enjoyed increasing growth in GDP (Figure 3.5).

Wages are also shown to have grown more in countries that have become more globalized (Figure 3.6). This reflects the relocation of manufacturing and other labour-intensive jobs from high- to low- and middle-income countries (e.g. footwear and clothing, toys, electronics, automobiles). This suggests that workers in more globalized countries are also benefiting from economic growth. An update of this work by Dollar et al. (2013) reasserts that 'growth still is good for the poor'. They write that 'we can expect economic growth to lift people out of poverty and lead to shared prosperity on average. The result also helps us understand how the rapid growth in the developing world in recent decades has led to such dramatic poverty reduction' (Dollar et al. 2013: 17).

In stark contrast to globalists is the so-called 'anti-globalization' movement, a diverse collection of interest groups that oppose current forms of economic globalization. It is more

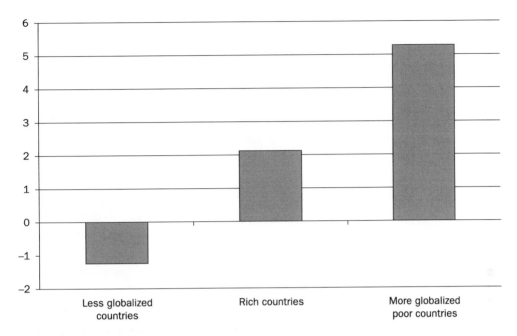

Figure 3.4 Percentage growth of GDP and degree of globalization

Source: Dollar and Kraay (2001)

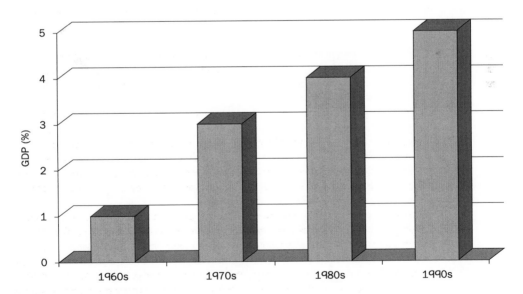

Figure 3.5 Per capita growth for more globalized countries

Source: Dollar and Kraay (2001)

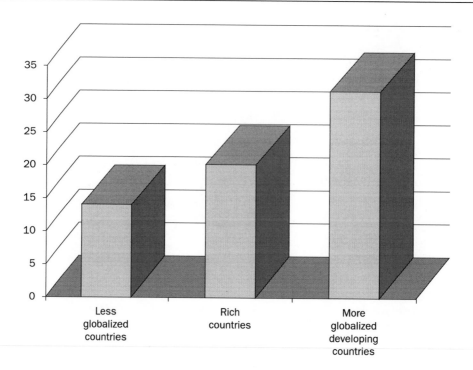

Figure 3.6 Wage growth by degree of globalization

Source: World Bank (2002)

accurate to describe this group as anti-Washington Consensus, rather than globalization *per se*. They argue that contemporary globalization is:

• increasing poverty;
• widening socioeconomic inequalities within and between countries;
• creating greater job insecurity;
• weakening workers' rights;
• undermining social welfare and environmental protection; and
• weakening democracy by enabling a global ruling class to act without sufficient transparency and accountability.

Many groups seeking to redirect economic globalization to alleviate poverty, achieve social justice, and ensure sustainable growth cite statistical evidence of the adverse impacts of recent trends. One measure is the Gini coefficient, which measures inequality within and between countries and is generally seen to be a truer measure of inequality within countries than GDP per capita. It is estimated that, between the 1950s and 1990s, 48 countries saw a rise in inequality (half the world's population), nine had less inequality, and 16 showed no trend (Table 3.5).

There is also concern about the social consequences of the so-called 'race to the bottom'. The greater ease by which capital can flow around the world means TNCs seek the most profitable locations in which to invest. This can mean investing in countries offering relatively cheap sources of inputs (including labour), and favourable tax and regulatory

Table 3.5 Trends in inequality, 1950s to 1990s

Trend in inequality	Number of countries	% of world population
Rising	48	47
Falling	9	4
No trend	16	29

Source: Cornia (2001).

policies. Countries competing to attract foreign direct investment are tempted to relax health and safety regulations for workers, environmental standards, and tax rates. For many workers in the global economy, this can mean lower wages and unsafe working conditions.

Shiva (in Mander 2000) writes that 'Globalisation of the economy is a new kind of colonialism visited upon poor countries and the poor in rich countries.' This appears to be supported by the proliferation of 'sweatshops' worldwide, as countries seek to increase their global competitiveness by reducing production costs. The working conditions of factories around the world have attracted negative public attention:

- In April 2013, more than 1100 people died and 2500 were injured in the collapse of a crowded and unsafe commercial building in Dhaka, Bangladesh. The building housed thousands of low-paid garment workers producing goods for overseas markets.
- The economic miracle in China has been accompanied by reports that forced and child labour has been used to supply the labour force. In 2010, Foxconn estimated that 150,000 of its workforce are students, including 28,000 'interns'. The company is the largest supplier to Apple and a major supplier to Sony.
- It was reported that 70 per cent of the staff at a Honda gearbox factory were from secondary schools. Many work long hours for low pay in unsafe conditions under coercive management (Chakrabortty 2013).

The apparent contradiction in data by globalists and its critics can easily confuse. Is globalization resulting in increased growth or reduced incomes? Is the developing world benefiting from economic globalization or becoming ever poorer? With the exception of the most hardened globalists, and most radical anti-globalization activists, what is increasingly clear is that globalization is creating patterns of winners and losers that cut across national borders. There is a need to tease apart aggregated datasets and to determine who are the specific winners and losers across a global economy. Population groups within and across countries need to be considered in terms of variations in total wealth, income distribution, resources, human capital, geography, infrastructure, and so on. No one policy, such as full-scale trade liberalization or privatization of state-owned industries, is suitable for all sectors in all countries. This was the approach of SAPs, which, while bringing some benefits to some populations, proved harmful for others. Moreover, understanding the health impacts of globalization requires recognition that the playing field is far from level. Economic globalization brings more benefits to those who are educated, have access to the information superhighway, have secure employment, and are relatively mobile. For others, policy measures are needed to remedy these disadvantages.

The work of Milanovic (1999) on household survey data is useful in this respect. He analysed the impacts of trade liberalization on income distribution within rich and poor countries. This means looking at not only rich and poor countries in aggregate, but also at rich and poor households within different countries. Analysing the impact of openness and foreign direct investment as a share of a country's GDP on the relative income of both the lowest and highest deciles (10%) of the population, he found that, in low-income countries, economic globalization tends to benefit the well-off. In middle-income countries (e.g. Colombia, Czech Republic, Malaysia), the incomes of the poor and middle class rise relative to the well-off. This is attributed to the availability of basic education, which enables more people to participate in the changing economy. He concludes that '[o]nly when at least basic education becomes the norm, can even the poor deciles share benefits of increased labour demand; then inequality falls' (Milanovic 1999).

In summary, the greatest challenge for economic globalization is to improve the current balance and distribution among those who gain from globalization and those who lose. Further research and policy responses are needed to identify and support those most unduly disadvantaged by the changes taking place, including wider environmental changes (further discussed in Chapter 13). Measures are needed to mitigate adverse impacts, and enable people to gain a fair share of the benefits from economic globalization.

✐ Activity 3.3

Economic globalization is prompting diverse, and often polarized, views on whether it is having positive or negative impacts on societies worldwide. Read the following four quotes about economic globalization:

Globalization and free trade do spur economic growth, and they lead to lower prices on many goods.

Robert Reich, former US Secretary of Labor (92Y Online 2005)

Globalization creates economic policies where the transnationals lord over us, and the result is misery and unemployment.

Evo Morales, President of Bolivia (Worley et al. 2013)

Globalization has created this interlocking fragility. At no time in the history of the universe has the cancellation of a Christmas order in New York meant layoffs in China.

Nassim Nicholas Taleb, financial trader (*The Washington Post* 2009)

Well, we see an increasingly weaker labor movement as a result of the overall assault on the labor movement and as a result of the globalization of capital.

Angela Davis, University of California, Santa Cruz (Frontline 1997)

For each quote, identify who is seen by the speaker as positively and/or negatively impacted by economic globalization.

1 To what extent do you agree with each of these quotes?
2 What consequences for health might be related to these impacts?

Feedback

You will have identified that Robert Reich identifies the benefactors from economic globalization to be consumers, largely in high-income countries, who benefit from lower cost goods and services. Morales laments the loss of power by low- and middle-income countries in a world where large corporations are increasingly dominant. The winners are the corporations and the losers are the countries that do not have equivalent economic power. Taleb refers to the capacity of consumers and markets in high-income countries to have a more direct link to producers, but that the impact of such a market means greater vulnerability of workers in the factories that produce such consumer goods. Davis similarly refers to non-unionized labour as vulnerable to the whims of the global economy, which benefit from greater mobility.

Summary

Globalization is most frequently associated with the changes emerging from economic globalization, which are impacting on societies across the world. The growth and spread of the global economy (trade and finance) are likely to continue apace, creating new opportunities and risks for health. In Chapter 8, we consider in greater detail the health implications of trade liberalization under the World Trade Organization.

Note

1 The special drawing right (SDR) is an international reserve asset, created by the IMF in 1969, to supplement its member states' official reserves. Its value is based on a basket of four key international currencies. SDRs can be exchanged for freely usable currencies.

References

BIS (2013) *BIS Quarterly Review, December 2013* [http://www.bis.org/publ/qtrpdf/r_qt1312.htm].

Carroll, P. and Kellow, A. (2011) *The OECD: A Study of Organisational Adaptation*. Cheltenham: Edward Elgar.

Chakrabortty, A. (2013) The woman who nearly dies making your iPad, *The Guardian*, Monday 5 August.

Christian Aid (2002) *World Social Forum 31 January–5 February 2002* [http://www.christian-aid.org.uk/wefwsf/wsf.htm].

Cornia, G.A. (2001) Globalization and health: results and options, *Bulletin of the World Health Organization*, 79 (9): 834–41.

Cullen, J.B. and Praveen Parboteeah, K. (2013) *Multinational Management*. Mason, OH: Cengage Learning.

Dollar, D., Kleineberg, T. and Kraay, A. (2013) Growth still is good for the poor. World Bank Policy Research Working Papers. Washington, DC: The World Bank [http://elibrary.worldbank.org/doi/pdf/10.1596/1813-9450-6568].

Dollar, D. and Kraay, A. (2001) Growth is good for the poor. World Bank Policy Research Department Working Paper No. 2587. Washington, DC: World Bank [http://www.worldbank.org/research/growth].

Editors (2013) *Horse-meat scandal exposes weakness in global food chain*, 24 March [http://www.bloomberg.com/news/2013-03-24/horse-meat-scandal-exposes-weakness-in-global-food-chain.html].

Falk, R. (1999) *Predatory Globalization: A Critique*. London: Polity Press.

Frontline (1997) *The Two Nations of Black America: An Interview with Angela Davis*. Public Broadcasting Station, 1997 [http://www.pbs.org/wgbh/pages/frontline/shows/race/interviews/davis.html].

Gabel, M. and Bruner, H. (2003) *An Atlas of the Multinational Corporation*. New York: The New Press.

Hajnal, P.I. (2007) Can civil society influence G8 accountability? Working Paper. Coventry: Centre for the Study of Globalisation and Regionalisation, University of Warwick [http://wrap.warwick.ac.uk/1873/].

IMF (2001) Refocusing IMF conditionality, *Finance & Development: A Quarterly Magazine of the IMF*, 38 (4).

Lal, D. (2006) *Reviving the Invisible Hand: The Case for Classical Liberalism in the Twenty-First Century*. Princeton, NJ: Princeton University Press.

Longworth, R. (1998) *Global Squeeze: The Coming Crisis for First-World Nations*. Chicago, IL: Contemporary Books.

Lugella, J. (1995) The impact of structural adjustment policies on women's and children's health in Tanzania, *Review of African Political Economy*, 22 (63): 43–53.

Mander, J. (2000) Corporate colonialism, *Resurgence* 179 [http://resurgence.gn.apc.org/articles/mander.htm].

Martin, H. and Schuman, H. (1997) *The Global Trap: Globalisation and the Assault on Democracy and Prosperity*. London: Pluto Press.

Milanovic, B. (1999) True world income distribution, 1988 and 1993: first calculations, based on household surveys alone. Poverty Working Paper No. 2244. Washington, DC: World Bank [http://ideas.repec.org/p/wbk/wbrwps/2244.html].

OECD (1960) *Convention on the Organization for Economic Cooperation and Development* [http://www.oecd.org/general/conventionontheorganisationforeconomicco-operationanddevelopment.htm].

OECD (n.d.) *Our mission* [http://www.oecd.org/about/].

Peabody, J. (1996) Economic reform and health sector policy: lessons from structural adjustment programs, *Social Science and Medicine*, 43 (5): 823–35.

Scholte, J.A. (2000) What is 'global' about globalization?, in J.A. Scholte (ed.) *Globalization: A Critical Introduction*, pp. 41–61. London: Macmillan.

Scrace, M. (2006) Cholera in the Mdletsheni Tribal Authority, *Journal of Rural and Tropical Public Health*, 5: 70–8.

Smith, G. (2011) *G7 to G8 to G20: Evolution in global governance*, CIGI G20 Papers No. 6, May. Waterloo, ON: The Centre for International Governance Innovation [http://www.cigionline.org/sites/default/files/G20No6.pdf].

The G8 Research Group (2012) G8 Information Centre. Toronto, ON: The G8 Research Group, University of Toronto [http://www.g8.utoronto.ca/evaluations/].

The G20 Research Group (2010) *What is the G20?* G20 Information Centre. Toronto, ON: The G20 Research Group, University of Toronto [http://www.g20.utoronto.ca/g20whatisit.html; accessed 4 July 2014].

The Washington Post (2009) A conversation with Nassim Nicholas Taleb, *The Washington Post*, 15 March 2009 [http://www.washingtonpost.com/wp-dyn/content/article/2009/03/12/AR2009031202181_pf.html].

UNCTAD (2012) *World Investment Report 2012* [http://unctad.org/en/PublicationsLibrary/wir2012_embargoed_en.pdf].

Werner, D. and Sanders, D. (1997) *Questioning the Solution: The Politics of Primary Health Care and Child Survival*. Palo Alto, CA: Health Rights.

Williamson, J. (1990) *Latin American Adjustment: How Much Has Happened?* Washington, DC: Institute for International Economics.

World Bank (2002) *Globalization, Growth and Poverty*. World Bank Policy Research Report. Washington, DC: World Bank.

World Economic Forum (n.d.) *World Economic Forum* [http://www.linkedin.com/company/world-economic-forum].

World Social Forum (2001) *Principle Charter*, Porto Alegre [http://www2.portoalegre.rs.gov.br/fsm2013_ing/default.php?p_secao=5].

Worley, C.G., Mirvis, P.H., Mohrman, S.A. and Shani, A.B. (2013) *Building Networks and Partnerships for Sustainability*. Bingley, UK: Emerald Group Publishing.

92Y Online. An interview with Robert Reich, New York, 2005 [http://blog.92y.org/index.php/item/robert_reich/].

Global health and governance

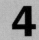

4

Preslava Stoeva, Johanna Hanefeld and Benjamin Hawkins

Overview

In this chapter, we will focus on the importance of governance to the pursuit of public health in the era of globalization. The chapter defines governance and provides a historical overview of how governance activities for public health have changed. While chapters 5–7 set out the different groups of key actors in global health governance and global governance for health, this chapter provides a framework for analysing and understanding the different health issues explored throughout the remainder of this book. It also provides an introduction to the politics of global health.

Learning objectives

After working through this chapter, you will be able to:

- define governance and distinguish it from government
- identify different levels of governance important for health
- describe how health governance has developed historically
- understand how and why health governance has changed
- relate governance frameworks to other issues in global health addressed in this book
- consider problems that confront the new governance context for health

Key terms

Governance: The process of governing, or of controlling, managing or regulating the affairs of some entity.

Government: The institutions and procedures for making and enforcing rules and other collective decisions within a sovereign state. This is a narrower concept than the state, which may also include the judiciary, military, and religious bodies.

Global governance: The sum of the many ways individuals and institutions, both public and private, manage their common affairs. Global governance is a continuing process through which conflicting or diverse interests may be accommodated and cooperative action may be taken. It includes formal as well as informal arrangements that people and institutions have agreed to or perceive to be in their interest (Commission on Global Governance 1995: 2).

Global governance for health: Governance efforts of all actors, both health and non-health, that aim to promote and protect health. This term is often used interchangeably with global health governance, but really emphasizes the whole-of-government and whole-of-society approach to health (i.e. it includes the contribution and activities of non-health sectors in health).

Global health governance: Governance among states and non-state actors in the field of health working to protect and promote health.

Horizontal governance: Governance by means of cooperation between sovereign states or units with commensurate power and authority.

Human right to health: The right of individuals to the highest attainable standard of health.

International governance: The process of governing the relations between states that involves only the states and inter-governmental organizations as relevant actors.

Public–private partnerships: Formal or informal joint endeavours involving state and non-state (both civil society and corporate) actors typically focused on a particular health policy issue or problem.

Vertical governance: Governance premised on hierarchical power relations, usually classified as 'top-down', that involves state and non-state actors above and below the sovereign state. For example, in certain areas of law within the European Union, where the EU sets standards for national legislation across all member states, or in a federal system, such as the United States.

Sovereignty: Supreme, exclusive power over the territory and people of a state, including a legal right to non-intervention in the internal and external affairs of that state.

Global health and governance

As set out in Chapter 1, global health has changed rapidly and significantly over the past two decades and is now seen as a major issue in world politics. As most health threats transcend borders and are influenced by factors that lie beyond the control of individual states, such as the environment, migration, and trade, it is often through global organizations (e.g. the World Health Organization) that they are addressed. While there are many definitions, the notion of governance refers to the ways in which society organizes and collectively manages its affairs. Governance is also often seen as incorporating the function of stewardship. At national level, the state is a key actor in governance, in the organization of different actors, and in the way policy responses to specific issues, such as health, are organized.

In global health, governance is distinct from that at national level as there is no global government. Rather, there is a myriad of actors, of which states are one, working on a wide range of issues but with no clear hierarchy except for the sovereignty of states. One of the features of global health and its governance over the past twenty years has been the proliferation of a wide range of state and non-state actors. This includes states who may seek to address transnational health concerns, such as avian influenza, to protect their population, or address an issue such as child malnutrition as part of a global solidarity agenda. States may become global health actors in their own right, or they may seek to pursue these issues through multilateral organizations, such as the WHO or UNICEF. The number of non-state actors has also increased over the past twenty years, including an increase in non-governmental organizations, public–private partnerships such as the Global Fund to Fight AIDS, Tuberculosis and Malaria, and private foundations like the Bill and Melinda Gates Foundation. These are discussed further in Chapter 7.

The impact of non-health factors on health, such as education and employment, is increasingly recognized, as are the unintended consequences of areas such as trade and security. This has further extended the scope and number of actors and organizations working on health-related issues. In the absence of one clear authority in global health, coordination between these different organizations, the mechanisms through which they interact and work together (i.e. the *governance* of global health), have become important to understanding global health.

Governance and government

Many contemporary political debates, including those in the field of global health, refer not to governments but to the process of governance. This shift in terminology reflects the evolving status of state governments in policy-making at both the national and global level within the context of globalization (see Chapter 5). To a certain degree, the concept of governance implies a weakening of the state as a policy actor as new policy actors emerge. The concept is particularly apt within the context of global (as opposed to international) health policy due to the conditions of 'anarchy', which determines the international sphere (i.e. the absence of an overarching power – or world government – to make and enforce laws). This requires forms of governance based on cooperation and coordination as opposed to regulation and enforcement, which characterize hierarchical forms of government at the national level. Examples of governance arrangements may include public–private partnerships, outsourcing, and private finance initiatives, which are widespread within the field of (global) health policy.

It is important to note that these categories, while useful for our understanding and analysis of governance, are artificial. Governance usually happens simultaneously at more than one level; segregating these provides an opportunity to study the behaviour of different actors and the process, dynamics, and outcomes of interactions and negotiations.

Continuity and change in global health governance

Concerted efforts by governing political authorities to deal with threats to population health, particularly infectious diseases, date back at least to the fourteenth-century Italian city-states (Liverani and Coker 2012). While the nature and scope of political authority have changed significantly in the intervening centuries, the task of protecting populations from external health-related threats has persisted on government agendas. However, governments are not the only actors involved in global health governance. This section will explore the changes and continuities in governance actors and processes related to public health across borders, from a historical perspective. Accounts of global health governance often focus on examining the role of states and the World Health Organization, missing out a much richer governance landscape, which holds clues about the current form of the system of governance, as well as contemporary policy preferences and priorities. We argue that there has been much continuity in patterns of cross-border health governance since the nineteenth century, despite changes in the disciplinary terminology and the emergence of new actors in health, such as the increasingly important role of the World Bank, or the OECD as discussed in Chapter 3.

State relations

States are the building blocks of the contemporary international system. Human communities evolved over time and the dominant form of organization for more than a century has been the sovereign state. Sovereignty is the exclusive right of states to be free from intervention in their internal or external affairs. The concept of sovereignty was established by the Treaty of Westphalia (1648), which ended the Thirty Years War (1618–48), a war that devastated much of Christian Europe in the aftermath of the Reformation and the split in the Church. The treaty was seen to secularize politics, by separating the state from the Church and declaring the absolute power of the sovereign within his or her territory. The sovereign was therefore free to adopt whatever religious or political system he or she deemed suitable. The notion that the sovereign is not subject to any higher authority in his or her internal and external relations remains one of the fundamental principles of international politics to the present day. Sovereignty further guarantees the legal equality of states. Collectively states are the only actors that can create norms, rules, and regulations to govern their conduct and interactions with other states and intergovernmental organizations (IGOs). Such rules, norms, and regulations form the body of public international law.

State relations are therefore premised on a conjunction of equal status but unequal power (Jackson 2006: 36–7), which can be a pre-condition for insecurity and conflict. State relations take place in the context of an *anarchic* international system, where no higher political authority than the sovereign state exists. As a result, scholars of international relations argue that each state has to rely on self-help and the pursuit of power, which guarantee its ability to protect and defend its people, territory, resources, and values from external intrusion. Recognized states are therefore seen to possess 'legitimate authority' to declare war, to enter into bilateral or multilateral agreements, and to create international legal norms. States are free to participate in international governance in a manner and to the extent to which they see fit. In this volatile context of international politics and limited rules, international scholars have argued, promises of cooperation could be broken without consequence and states were more likely to be involved in conflict than commit to cooperation (Morgenthau 1993). This was particularly so in the realm of 'high politics', which included defence and security. While scholars admitted some cooperation was possible in areas of 'low politics', as these were not of strategic significance, it would be dominated by and be conducted largely in the interest of the most powerful states.

In contemporary state relations, conflict and cooperation continue to be defining features. National security politics and state foreign policies show clear signs of persistent state concerns with the proliferation of weapons, conflict, instability, and increasingly the threat posed by international terrorism. International cooperation in international relations is often described as limited, difficult, and complicated by various intervening factors. These include national interests, poverty and unequal economic development, economic crises affecting states differently, cultural differences, and differences in political systems to name just a few. This is despite the intensifying of economic and social globalization described in Chapters 1 and 2, which have led to greater interaction between people across borders. Cooperation can be bilateral or multilateral. Bilateral cooperation takes place between two states, while multilateral cooperation can be regional, international, multi-issue or issue-specific. The most well-known contemporary example of multi-issue international cooperation is the United Nations, which will be discussed in greater detail later on in this chapter.

Bilateral and multilateral cooperation on health issues has a fairly extensive history, which began when states were affected by the cross-border spread of communicable diseases through international trade. The intensification of international trade and travel, particularly in the late twentieth century, increased the amount and variety of health-related risks and threats faced by states. It became obvious that some states were better equipped to address these, while others relied more extensively on international cooperation and support. Growing disparities in the ability of states to respond to health challenges became even more apparent following the economic crisis of the early 1970s, which highlighted the stark inequalities in economic development and wealth accumulation between North and South. The economies of the so-called 'Third World' countries were predominantly weak, dependent on trade with the richer economies of the 'First World' and on international borrowing, and negatively affected by an inequitable distribution of resources. While economic growth has occurred since the 1970s, such growth has become increasingly unequal with inequalities within as well as between countries (WHO 2008). These inequalities have been perhaps most visible in health, with people in low-income countries often experiencing worse health and a shorter life than those in middle- and high-income countries. Simultaneously, within countries, people facing marginalization or exclusion in other areas commonly also have the worst health. An example of this is maternal mortality, with most maternal deaths occurring in low-income countries, and within countries rates of maternal mortality are often much higher in minorities, for example, the indigenous populations in South America (Backman et al. 2008).

As a result of these inequities, the pursuit of common, global health goals has since appeared more as a chimera than a pragmatic possibility. Efforts to intensify international cooperation and assistance have increased in the early twenty-first century, evidenced by the commitment of states to the Millennium Development Goals – three of which focus explicitly on health. The challenges faced in global health politics are multiple and complex, as this chapter seeks to demonstrate.

✏ Activity 4.1

Think about a health issue such as maternal mortality, HIV/AIDS or a non-communicable disease in the country and region you are in. Try to identify who is affected by the issue and if this is equally distributed within your country or region, or if particular sections of the population are more affected than others.

Feedback

You will likely find that some groups or parts of the population are more affected than others (i.e. face a greater burden of disease). The inequities are also likely to have grown over the past decades and often link to other factors, such as poverty, employment status or gender. This highlights the uneven growth since the 1970s and the extent to which other sectors are important to health.

Since the end of the Cold War in 1989, the scope of state cooperation through bilateral and multilateral agreements as well as through inter-governmental organizations (both regional and global) has intensified. As set out in Chapter 1, as part of the processes of globalization the volume of international trade, travel, and communications has increased dramatically. The likelihood of an all-out nuclear war decreased in the aftermath of the diffused super-power rivalry between the United States and the Soviet Union. Many scholars have since questioned the relevance of the high/low politics classification, arguing that many issues formerly considered as part of the low politics agenda have implications for the strategic interests of states, as well as for the maintenance of national and international security. Others have challenged the continued primacy of the state in international politics:

> where states were once the masters of markets, now it is the markets which, on many crucial issues, are the masters over the governments of states . . . the declining authority of states is reflected in a growing diffusion of authority to other institutions and associations, and to local and regional bodies, and in a growing asymmetry between the larger states with structural power and weaker ones without it.
>
> (Strange 1996: 69)

Perhaps the most important change in contemporary politics has been the desire to expand the meaning of the concept of sovereignty. The concept of *Responsibility to Protect* (R2P), proposed at the UN Summit in 2005, deems that apart from rights, states have responsibilities towards their citizens, upon which their right to non-intervention is conditional. This marked an important development in inter-state relations, as it highlights the contingency of a state's responsibility towards its citizens and its sovereignty (UNGA 2005).

Multilateral cooperation

The earliest forms of state cooperation in health governance took place in a regional context. While regional cooperation differed widely, its defining characteristics included geographical proximity and the desire of neighbouring states to achieve common aims. Some of the oldest regional health organizations include the Conseil supérieur de Santé de Constantinople, Ottoman Empire (1830s), the Conseil Sanitaire de Tanger, Morocco (1840), the Egyptian Quarantine Board established in Alexandria (1843), which later became the regional epidemiological bureau of the Office International d'Hygiène Publique, and the Conseil Sanitaire de l'Empire, set up by the Shah of Persia (1867) (Lee 2009: 3). All of these organizations sought through various means to control the spread of infectious diseases related to international trade and travel. Efforts were primarily focused on the control of the spread of infectious diseases, including cholera and plague, and the method of choice was quarantine, which refers to a period or place of isolation in which people or animals that have arrived from elsewhere or have been exposed to infectious or contagious disease are placed.

In the spirit of multilateral diplomacy, fourteen International Sanitary Conferences took place in Europe between 1851 and 1938. Convened by the Government of France, they sought to establish agreed standards on quarantine regulations, so that these did not interfere with the growing volumes of international trade and travel, and to coordinate international efforts. Four International Sanitary Conventions were agreed between 1892 and 1903. These significant developments are indeed the early forms of what we refer to in contemporary terms as global health governance.

The Pan-American Sanitary Bureau (PASB) was established in 1902, in the aftermath of the first few International Sanitary Conferences (ISCs). It is the predecessor of the Pan American Health Organization (PAHO), which today serves as the regional office of the World Health Organization for the Americas. The PASB was set up in part because there was a strong feeling that the ISCs catered primarily to the needs and interests of European states (Borowy 2010; Lee 2009: 4). The organization was small and worked with limited resources, but laid the foundations of important future developments – such as cross-border data collection, and the exchange and sharing of information. There are three distinct characteristics of the early work of PAHO: the dominance of the United States in the organization in its early years, the desire to seek local solutions for local problems, and the introduction of the 'social medicine' approach, which emphasizes the social and economic determinants of specific population health problems (Fee and Brown 2002: 1889). While these idiosyncrasies are generated by the specific political and economic realities in the Americas, the desire of the United States to play a leading role in regional and international cooperation (with a short relapse during the years of American isolationism in the 1930s and early 1940s) has defined many aspects of international politics and some features of inter-governmental organizations.

In 1907, the Office International d'Hygiène Publique (OIHP) was established in Paris. European states used the organization to collect and share information and epidemiological data and to pursue a collective response to the threats of cholera, the plague, and yellow fever, which were spread through the intensifying international trade and travel (Borowy 2010). The OIHP has since been incorporated in the administrative mechanisms of the World Health Organization (WHO).

Specialized regional health organizations no longer exist, but decision-making on various aspects of public health continues to take place in the context of some regional organizations such as the EU and ASEAN, as well as through the regional offices of the WHO.

Inter-governmental organizations

Multilateral state cooperation beyond regional relations has been steadily increasing with the evolution of the means of transportation and communication technologies. The practice of multilateral diplomacy of the sixteenth and seventeenth centuries has been replaced by more permanent arrangements in the form of inter-governmental organizations. An inter-governmental organization (IGO) is composed primarily of sovereign states (three or more), is created through a written agreement, and has a permanent secretariat (Union of International Associations). While this sub-section discusses international IGOs, it is worth noting that regional organizations are also a form of IGO.

States tend to form international governmental organizations to reduce the transaction costs of their cooperation, to achieve foreign policy aims, to promote cooperation and security, to achieve goals that they cannot attain on their own, as well as to deal with and regulate intensifying cross-border relations (Keohane and Nye 1977). The number of IGOs created by states has grown exponentially from a handful at the start of the nineteenth century to an estimated 238 in 2004 (Armstrong et al. 2004; Boli and Thomas 1999). The downside of such growth is the development of competition between organizations not only for resources but also for leadership on specific issues. The expanding mandates of different organizations also lead to overlap in activities with little coordination. Barnett and Finnemore (2004) argue that significant changes occur in IGOs over time, as they develop their bureaucratic rational legal authority, which allows them to broaden their mandates and expertise and gain a level of decision-making autonomy. Barnett and Finnemore (2004: 7) use the examples of the International Monetary Fund, the UN High Commissioner for Refugees, and the peacekeeping culture in the United Nations to demonstrate how 'IOs help determine the kind of world that is to be governed and set the agenda for global governance', thus claiming a far more influential role for these actors than previously acknowledged. Such proliferation of IGOs has added to the complexity of global governance.

The first dedicated international health organization was set up under the first multilateral, multi-issue inter-governmental organization – the League of Nations. The League of Nations was established as part of the peace settlement of the First World War in 1920 to promote international cooperation, transparency in state relations, and to avoid another Great War. The League of Nations Health Organization (LNHO) was set up in 1922 to seek cooperation even with governments who were not members of the League (e.g. Germany, the USA, the USSR). This is the precursor of later attempts towards more inclusive international cooperation, promoted by the United Nations. The driving forces behind the LNHO were the colonial powers and members – Britain, France, Belgium, Italy, and Spain. The League's membership created specific power dynamics, which had an impact on the agenda and priorities of the organization, as discussed by Borowy (2010). The organization's Health Section acted as a link between national health administrations, promoting technical assistance between governments and advising the Health Council and the League's Assembly on questions of international public health.

The League of Nations was disbanded at the start of the Second World War – the very development it was set up to prevent. The Second World War was the single most devastating conflict that the world had seen. Even before it had come to an end, President Roosevelt and Prime Minister Churchill pledged to work closely to develop better forms of international cooperation by signing the Atlantic Charter (1941), Clause 6 of which read: 'After the final destruction of Nazi tyranny [we] hope to see established a peace which will afford to all nations the means of dwelling in safety within their own boundaries, and which will afford assurance that all the men in all the lands may live out their lives in freedom from fear and want' (UN n.d.). The Atlantic Charter (1941) was the predecessor of the Declaration of the United Nations (1942), which became the foundation of the United Nations Charter, signed in 1945 at the San Francisco Conference, establishing the Organization of the United Nations. The World Health Organization came into existence shortly after in 1948, incorporating the League of Nations Health Organization, the Office International d'Hygiène Publique, and the Pan-American Health Bureau, continuing the tradition of inclusivity, representation, and inter-governmental cooperation in health governance. The WHO Constitution was adopted at the International Health Conference, held in New York in 1946, and was signed by the representatives of the 61 states present at the conference. The constitution defined health as 'a state of complete physical, mental and social well-being, and not merely the absence of disease or infirmity'. It also stipulated that '[t]he enjoyment of the highest attainable standard of health is one of the fundamental rights of every human being, without distinction of race, religion, political belief, economic or social condition' (WHO 1948).

In 2014, WHO had 194 member states, each of which has one vote in the World Health Assembly – the WHO's main decision-making body, which meets once a year to determine the strategic direction and policies of the organization. The WHO's regional structure – of six regional offices and many country offices – is a historical legacy, since the WHO absorbed existing regional organizations. Chapter 5 discusses the organization's role in greater detail.

While the WHO is the dedicated agency of the UN to address issues of health, it is not the only one involved in governance for health. Questions of health are intertwined with issues of human rights, labour laws, economic development, and poverty alleviation, and more recently with security (both human and state) and environmental change and degradation. The WHO is meant to be the leading health IGO, but the World Bank has for some time played a large part in health internationally, while the United Nations Development Programme, the International Labour Organization, the World Trade Organization, and UNAIDS have all been involved with different aspects of global health governance, which has not always complemented the work of the WHO. This has generated tensions in the field of global health governance, questions about its future, and debates about the need to reform the WHO or seek a stronger, more effective leader in the field of health politics. Others have proposed a framework convention on global health that would see responsibilities and remit clearly divided between international organizations. This refers to both those organizations in the field of health and others such as the G8 or the G20, discussed in Chapter 3, whose work is outside the remit of health, but nonetheless vitally important to health itself.

Non-governmental organizations and global health governance

As pointed out at the start of this chapter, states and inter-governmental organizations are not the only actors that influence health politics and governance. While the idiosyncrasies of the nature of the involvement of NGOs, civil society, and private and corporate actors in global health governance will be explored in greater detail in Chapters 6 and 7, we wish to demonstrate here the continuities and changes of this involvement from a historic perspective.

Civil society, humanitarian and philanthropic organizations developed alongside states and inter-governmental organizations in the eighteenth and nineteenth centuries. One of the most recognizable private transnational organizations – the International Committee of the Red Cross (ICRC) – was set up in 1863 as the International Committee to Aid the Military Wounded, by a group of five individuals: Henry Dunant, a Swiss banker, Gustave Moynier, a Swiss lawyer, General Dufour, commander of the Swiss Army and two physicians, Louis Appia and Theodore Maunoir. They were determined to create national relief societies, staffed by qualified volunteers to care for the wounded in wartime (Finnemore 1999: 154–5). The organization's initial scope of activity – assisting wounded soldiers in international war – has expanded to cover various aspects of humanitarian law (helping civilians, refugees, internally displaced persons, etc.) and even touches on some human rights issues that transcend conflict situations (Forsythe 2005: 2). The ICRC is the founding agency of the International Red Cross and the Red Crescent Movement, which further comprises the International Federation of Red Cross and Red Crescent Societies and 188 individual National Societies. Its mission is to 'alleviate human suffering, protect life and health, and uphold human dignity especially during armed conflicts and other emergencies' (ICRC 2013). The movement works closely with other non-governmental organizations and is funded largely by voluntary donations from national governments. The ICRC is on the one hand a unique type of organization due to its development, main characteristics, and unusual relationship with national governments, (Forsythe 2005), but on the other it is a typical example of a private transnational actor, unregulated by governments, which delivers health-related care and humanitarian assistance, in tandem with other NGOs such as Médecins Sans Frontières (MSF) and Oxfam, and strives to abide by the humanitarian principles of humanity, impartiality, neutrality, and independence.

The beginning of the twentieth century saw the emergence of an altogether different type of non-governmental entity – the philanthropic foundation, often linked to corporations or individuals from the corporate world. The Rockefeller Foundation was one of a number of private funds and foundations (including the Carnegie Foundation, Milbank Memorial Fund, and Sage Foundation), which provided finance for education, health, and biomedical research, both domestically in the United States and to developed and developing countries alike. Some of these actors will be discussed further in Chapter 7. It is important to note how deeply embedded they are in policy processes, and how long-lived this form of political influence is. The Rockefeller Foundation, for example, provided considerable financial support to the League of Nations Health Organization. Some scholars have argued that the foundation has primarily aimed to further American political and private corporate interests through its support for the League and through its own initiatives. These have included establishing training centres, schools of public health, education and research programmes in Europe (Weindling 1993), the Far East, and Latin America (Cueto 1997; Weindling 1995). For example, the Rockefeller Sanitary Commission for the Eradication of Hookworm Disease was established in 1909 to address hookworm disease in the southern states of the United States, where the Rockefellers had direct economic interests in the production of raw materials (Brown 1976: 898). Brown collected his materials from the archives of the foundations, including internal memos, correspondence, and reports and illuminates the intentions behind health-related investments – namely, 'to raise the productivity of the workers in underdeveloped countries . . . to reduce the cultural autonomy of these agrarian peoples . . . [and] to assuage hostility to the US and undermine goals of national economic and political independence' (Brown 1976: 900). Birn and Fee similarly observed that through its investment in the hookworm, yellow fever, and malaria campaigns, the Rockefeller Foundation prepared vast regions for investment and increased productivity. The Rockefeller Foundation chose its campaigns carefully to avoid campaigns that would be 'costly, overly complex, time-consuming, or distracting to its technically oriented public health model and its focused means of measuring success' (Birn and Fee 2013: 1618). The Rockefeller Foundation is credited with inventing the public–private partnership model, which is now common in global health, and with establishing a technically oriented approach to health emulated by other foundations, including the Bill and Melinda Gates Foundation.

Appraising the work of private philanthropic agencies in a critical manner presents some challenges – private donations and expert programmes contribute to improvements in the health of populations in different corners of the world, even if they are seen to have ulterior motives. Political or economic motives may be easier to ascribe than to verify, particularly when dealing with private actors, as there are no clear standards of accountability for such actors. Some of these criticisms may be equally valid in relation to non-governmental and civil society organizations, whose work is similarly not regulated by established standards of accountability.

The scope and scale of the activities of private, non-governmental organizations have expanded significantly since the start of the twentieth century. Contrary to popular expectations, this growth was not confined to the years following the end of the Cold War, even though the latter accelerated the already apparent trend towards civil activism and private action. While most of these organizations continue to focus on delivering humanitarian assistance, an increasing number are also being subcontracted to assist with the delivery of public health services in chronic conflict or post-conflict situations.

Activity 4.2

Think about a health issue you are working on, or have studied. List all the actors and organizations that you can think of working on the issue. What kinds of organizations are they?

Feedback

You may have listed state actors such as government ministries, regulatory bodies or government agencies. Your list of actors may also have included non-governmental organizations and partners from other countries. This mix of actors highlights both the continuity and the changes in global health governance, as well as the multitude of actors involved.

The politics of global health governance

The governance of global health is not only deeply political, it takes place in a complex context with changing characteristics and competing political priorities, scarce resources, and a profusion of public and private actors, as discussed above. In principle, the well-being and prosperity of citizens are the responsibility of sovereign states and attempts to interfere without the express consent of the home state can be viewed as hostile. There is a history of interpreting attempts by international actors to create or improve health systems and educate health professionals as amounting to the consolidation of colonial power and a reflection of imperial ambitions. This section will discuss what impact some key political and economic factors might have on the politics of global health governance.

Influence of the wider political context

The impact of the wider regional and global political context is important. Colonialism, war, the politics of ideological competition between East and West during the Cold War and the resulting nuclear proliferation, decolonization and national self-determination, the pursuit of human rights, all are significant developments and often shape aspects of regional and international politics. While sovereign states are equal in terms of legal status, they do not possess equal power, making some states more vulnerable or susceptible to the influence of and even coercion by more powerful states. The politics of power are at the heart of studies of international relations, which aim to understand the nature of power and its effects on global politics, the nature of the relations between states, the propensity of states to engage in conflict and cooperation, and so on. The governance of health policies is one aspect of global politics and it is governed to some degree by similar forces. At the same time, the nature of the threat posed by diseases and ill health, and the need for a collective response may in many situations spur international cooperation. Changes in attitudes and public opinion also affect the direction international politics and collective action can take.

For example, the invention of penicillin and vaccines in the early twentieth century generated a feeling of the invincibility of humanity and a general belief in the power of science to combat any and all diseases. The successful smallpox eradication campaign led by the WHO provided hope that societies across the world can eliminate or at least significantly decrease the burden of communicable diseases. This attitude was challenged in the 1980s and 1990s by the emergence of new challenges such as HIV and AIDS, as well as of multidrug-resistant forms of known infectious diseases, including tuberculosis. Reports by government agencies and independent think tanks in the United States in the mid-1990s began to talk about the new security threat posed by emerging and re-emerging communicable diseases. The aftermath of the Cold War also raised concerns about the safety of smallpox strands in the former Soviet Union and the progress of decommissioning chemical and biological weapons. The anthrax attacks in the aftermath of 9/11 and the Tokyo subway sarine gas attack raised fears of bioterrorism.

Issue interconnectedness

Global health is thus directly and indirectly influenced by decision-making and regulations in other spheres of policy-making. Examples include the impact of TRIPs and the General Agreement on Trade in Services (GATS). A global regime regulating intellectual property rights has a profound effect on the production and trade of drugs, access to drugs, the development of drugs for neglected diseases (which may not be of interest to pharmaceutical companies seeking the most profitable segments of the market), and the advertising of products such as alcohol and tobacco. Regulations of food safety standards can be simultaneously beneficial and detrimental to public health in low-income countries or even to poor sections of societies in middle- and high-income countries. There is an increasing demand for research into how changes in the global climate and environment might impact health. Such changes could threaten food production, but could also affect the spread of infectious diseases, access to clean water, or cause increased migration, exacerbating existing public health problems. The full impact of interrelated factors can be difficult to evaluate, partly due to the number of issues that are simultaneously debated at the international level, and partly due to the fact that developments in some areas may have unintended consequences for health. For this reason, scholars in the field of global health governance are advocating the development of more multi- and inter-disciplinary methods to develop a more comprehensive understanding of the way in which different policy fields are connected and affect each other.

✐ **Activity 4.3**

Can you think of a health issue or a disease outbreak in a country where responses have been shaped by political factors and considerations? What may these factors have been?

Feedback

Disease outbreaks take many different forms. Some, such as the SARS outbreak in 2003, may have economic consequences, which in turn may shape the response. For example, fewer people may travel to an area or trade may be affected. This could influence how a country or a group of countries reacts to such an outbreak. It may also affect whether countries react together, either through an international organization focused on health, such as the WHO, or through a trade body such as ASEAN or the

World Trade Organization. Note that some of the action will extend beyond traditional 'health' actors, highlighting both the extent to which health is now considered an issue of high politics and the importance of other sectors to health.

Summary

In this chapter, we have explored the history of health in international relations and chartered the rise of the current era of global health governance. Taking a historic perspective has allowed us to examine the extent to which commonalities persist as well as the factors which shape and influence global health.

A feature of the emerging global health governance reviewed is that, in spite of the range of actors and new methods of working, sovereign states have remained a fundamental unit within it. Different examples, including the TRIPs agreement, demonstrate two characteristics: (i) the persistence and continued importance of sovereign nation-states as actors in global health, and (ii) the extent to which policies and actions taken in global health reflect imbalances in power between different actors. Global health is clearly seen as an issue of 'high politics'; indeed, it is considered a security issue and its governance is characterized by corresponding complexity and competing agendas. Discussions around clarifying this new global health governance or global governance for health to ensure efficiency and fairness have included a focus on the role of WHO and the organization's reform process. Yet even reform proposals such as the Framework Convention for Global Health confirm the state as the central unit.

A further aspect that emerges clearly from this analysis is the extent to which health is interconnected with other issues and how much non-health actors and issues influence global health. Thus any efforts at global governance for health need to take account of and include these competing agendas. The following three chapters explore the roles and practices of key actors within global health governance and how these affect health and its governance.

References

Armstrong, D., Lloyd, L. and Redmond, J. (2004) *International Organisation in World Politics* (3rd revised edn). Basingstoke: Palgrave Macmillan.

Backman, G., Hunt, P., Khosla, R., Jaramillo-Strouss, C., Fikre, B.M., Rumble, C. et al. (2008) Health systems and the right to health: an assessment of 194 countries, *The Lancet*, 372 (9655): 2047–85.

Barnett, M. and Finnemore, M. (2004) *Rules for the World: International Organizations in Global Politics*. Ithaca, NY: Cornell University Press.

Birn, A.-E. and Fee, E. (2013) The Rockefeller Foundation and the international health agenda, *The Lancet*, 381 (9878): 1618–19.

Boli, J. and Thomas, G.M. (eds.) (1999) *Constructing World Culture: International Nongovernmental Organisations Since 1875*. Stanford, CA: Stanford University Press.

Borowy, I. (2010) The League of Nations Health Organisation: from European to global health governance?, in A. Andresen, W. Hubbard and T. Ryymin (eds.) *International and Local Approaches to Health and Health Care*. Bergen: University of Bergen.

Brown, E.R. (1976) Public health in imperialism: early Rockefeller programs at home and abroad, *American Journal of Public Health*, 66: 897–903.

Commission on Global Governance (1995) *Our Global Neighbourhood*. Oxford: Oxford University Press.

Cueto, M. (1997) Science under adversity: Latin American medical research and American private philanthropy, 1920–1960, *Minerva*, 35: 233–45.

Fee, E. and Brown, T.M. (2002) 100 years of the Pan American Health Organization, *American Journal of Public Health*, 92 (12): 1888–9.

Finnemore, M. (1999) The rules of war and wars of rules: the International Red Cross and the restraint of state violence, in J. Boli and G. Thomas (eds) *Constructing World Culture: International Nongovernmental Organisations Since 1875*. Stanford, CA: Stanford University Press.

Forsythe, D. (2005) *The Humanitarians: The International Committee of the Red Cross*. Cambridge: Cambridge University Press.

ICRC (2013) *The Movement*. Geneva: ICRC [http://www.icrc.org/eng/who-we-are/movement/overview-the-movement.htm].

Jackson, J.H. (2006) *Sovereignty, the WTO, and Changing Fundamentals of International Law*. Cambridge: Cambridge University Press.

Keohane, R.O. and Nye, J.S. (1977) *Power and Interdependence: World Politics in Transition*. Boston MA: Little, Brown.

Lee, K. (2009) *The World Health Organization (WHO)*. London: Routledge.

Liverani, M. and Coker, R. (2012) Protecting Europe from diseases: from the International Sanitary Conferences to the ECDC, *Journal of Health Politics, Policy and Law*, 37: 915–34.

Morgenthau, H.J. (1993) *Politics among Nations: The Struggle for Power and Peace* (7th edn). New York: McGraw-Hill.

Strange, S. (1996) *The Retreat of the State: The Diffusion of Power in the World Economy*. Cambridge: Cambridge University Press.

UN (n.d.) *History of the Charter of the United Nations* [http://www.un.org/en/aboutun/charter/history/atlantic.shtml, accessed 22 October 2013].

UNGA (2005) Outcome Resolution, UN World Summit 2005 UN A/RES/60/1, New York.

UNOG (n.d.) League of Nations: History, *Site of the Library and Archives of the United Nations Office in Geneva* [http://www.unog.ch/80256EE60057D930/(httpPages)/03F1E1DD124D3276C1256F32002EE3AB?, accessed 22 October 2013].

Weindling, P. (1993) Public health and political stabilisation: the Rockefeller Foundation in Central and Eastern Europe between the two World Wars, *Minerva*, 31: 253–67.

Weindling, P. (ed.) (1995) *International Health Organisations and Movements, 1918–1939*. Cambridge: Cambridge University Press.

WHO (1948) *Constitution of the World Health Organization* [http://www.who.int/governance/eb/who_constitution_en.pdf].

WHO (2001) *Declaration on the TRIPS Agreement and Public Health* [http://www.wto.org/english/thewto_e/minist_e/min01_e/mindecl_trips_e.htm].

WHO (2008) *Closing the Gap in a Generation*. Geneva: World Health Organization.

Globalization – the state, bilateral and multilateral cooperation

5

Benjamin Hawkins

Overview

In this chapter, we examine the consequences of globalization for the state as a political entity and highlight the crucial role played by the state within the structure of global health governance. For example, an appreciation of what the state is and how its role has evolved is crucial to understanding how international organizations function and the role played by different global health actors such as corporations and civil society organizations.

Learning objectives

After working through this chapter, you will be able to:

- differentiate between the role of the state in domestic and international affairs
- distinguish between bilateral and multilateral forms of cooperation in the context of globalization
- compare the role of the state with that of other key actors in global health policy
- evaluate the extent to which the state remains the predominant actor in global health

Key terms

Bilateral cooperation: The relationship, both formal and informal, between two states. This may be in the forms of officially codified and legally enforceable trade agreements or looser forms of engagement.

Multilateral cooperation: Relationships formed between multiple actors, often enshrined in international organizations such as the World Trade Organization.

The state: A nation or territory that constitutes an organized political community under a government. The term is often used to denote the government of a particular territory, especially in the context of international organizations and the discipline of international relations, which analyses political interactions between states.

> 🖊 **Activity 5.1**
>
> Drawing on what you have learned in previous chapters, think about the characteristics of the state as a political actor. List the roles of the state as a political actor in the field of health. When you have done this, try to come up with a definition of the state in one or two sentences. Compare your definition with the discussion of the state below.

The idea of the state

Within the fields of political science and political philosophy, attempts to theorize the role of the state and the limits of state power extend back to ancient Greece. Plato's *Republic*, for example, is an attempt to work out the ideal model for the state. These attempts continue up to the present day and are at the heart of some of the fiercest political and ideological debates in modern political discourse. In the USA, for example, the emergence of the Tea Party Movement is, at least in part, a reaction to what conservatives see as the state stepping beyond its constitutionally defined remit and into areas of citizens' lives in which it has no right to intervene.

Within contemporary debates, a distinction is drawn in the role of the state between the domestic and the international spheres. The so-called internal and external functions of the state are the objects of study of the fields of political science and international relations, respectively. Within these disciplines there are very different assumptions made about the role of the state and the ability of the state to govern effectively.

The state and domestic politics

Numerous attempts have been made to define, describe, and critique the role of the state within the domestic sphere. Within the field of *political philosophy*, thinkers such as Thomas Hobbes (1960) and John Locke (1988) have attempted to justify the existence of the state and to define the role it ought to play in the lives of the citizens it governs. Simplifying greatly, Hobbes' contention is that the state is necessary to regulate the interactions between individuals; to create an overarching authority which can regulate their behaviour and enforce laws. Without the state, Hobbes contends, men – and it was principally men Hobbes thought of at the time of writing – are engaged in a continuous state of conflict with one another: what he termed 'the war of all against all'. The role of the state is, therefore, to regulate these affairs to the benefit of all citizens.

Hobbes' ideas were developed further by Locke. He sought to clarify just how far the state may justifiably go in limiting the freedom of the individual in order to benefit the collective. Locke uses the idea of individual property rights to define the limits of state activity, but nevertheless sees a robust role for the state in guaranteeing the rights of the individual (including their property rights) and enforcing the rule of law. This has obvious implications for the right of the state to levy taxes and to redistribute wealth through the tax system and, as such, is at the heart of contemporary debates about the retrenchment of the welfare state in many countries.

Perhaps the most famous and often quoted definition of the role of the state is that of the German sociologist Max Weber (1972). Weber claimed that what differentiates the state from other political actors, what defines it as an entity, is that it has what Weber terms 'a monopoly over the legitimate use of violence'. That is, the state has the right to employ violence in order to enforce the rule of law and that its ability to do so is both legally inscribed and accepted by those it governs. In concrete terms, this means that while the state may use a variety of means to get citizens to comply with the law, such as fining them or forbidding them to enter certain places, it is able to use physical coercion to enforce the law by, for example, arresting somebody by placing them in jail or using electronic tagging devices to track their movements.

Within the field of *political science*, scholars have attempted to explain how the state functions and what the consequences of its activities are. The most celebrated contributions to this field of scholarship represent the broader approaches to the study of politics indicated in italics. Ralph Miliband (1969) offers a *Marxist* analysis of the state, which argues that the structures of the state serve the interests of the establishment and those who control capital at the expense of the majority of the citizenry. Robert Dahl (1961), by contrast, offers a *pluralist* account of the state in which he sees a multiplicity of actors competing for power and influence at different junctures of the state apparatus. The *institutionalist* account of the state found in the works of Theda Skocpol (1979) emphasizes the autonomy of state institutions – and the actors within these institutions – from other societal actors and social pressures exerted on the state. Consequently, given their privileged position within the state machinery, the preferences of certain actors and the cultures of particular institutions are able to exert significant influence over society.

The state in the international sphere

It is the activity of the state at the international level that is of most obvious relevance to the study of global health. While the role of the state in the international sphere differs greatly from its role within the domestic sphere, it has been the focus of no less scholarly attention. This section addresses the principal tenets of these approaches within the discipline of *International Relations* (IR). There are long-standing debates within IR between proponents of different theoretical approaches to the subject. While theoretical debates can seem disconnected from the reality on the ground that motivates many health policy actors, they offer an important means of analysing global health and how globalization affects health. If we are driven by a desire to improve health, it is crucial to diagnose the precise nature of the problem that confronts us. Different theories offer competing accounts of the problems we face, presenting equally different solutions to these problems. As such, the theoretical lens through which we examine health determines both the way we understand global health and the way we engage with concrete political issues in this context.

The principal difference in these theories centres on the role of the state in the international arena and how states respond to the condition of *anarchy*, which is the defining characteristic of international politics. The concept of anarchy refers to the absence of an overarching global authority to govern the relationship between states in the same way that the state acts as the ultimate authority governing the relations between individuals in the domestic sphere. This is of vital importance to debates in global health policy, as the types of policy solution that may be feasible in the domestic sphere under state governments, may not be possible at the global level. Thus, new forms of governance arrangement are needed that seek to coordinate state behaviour (and that of other policy actors) and aim to foster cooperation between states in different forms. Each of the theories set out below represents a broad tradition of thinking about international politics and shows that there are some differences of emphasis that exist between them. They offer different lenses through which to analyse and evaluate current debates in global health.

They provide a set of different lenses to examine some of the processes in global health governance discussed in the preceding chapter. The following sections seek to unpack some of their main assumptions and insights.

Realism

Realist scholars assume that states are the principal, if not the only, actors in the international sphere. States in turn are concerned primarily with their *survival* and *security*, and the role of state leaders is to pursue policies that will guarantee this. For realists, then, security is equated with state security. The anarchic nature of the international domain means that states must rely on themselves to guarantee their security. International institutions are unable to provide the guarantee of security that states require. In the field of trade, realists argue governments ought to intervene to support domestic industry and to promote the national economy.

In addition to security, realists place great emphasis on the concept of state sovereignty and the principle of non-intervention. These refer to the ability of states to govern their internal affairs free from interference by other states. The principle of non-intervention derives from the Treaty of Westphalia of 1648 from which many of the norms for the conduct of international diplomacy originate. Given the emphasis placed on sovereignty and non-intervention in the conduct of international relations since, realist scholars are sceptical about the right of international organizations to intervene in the internal affairs of a state, as well the effectiveness of these organizations in regulating inter-state relations. For example, does the World Health Organization (WHO) have the right to demand countries disclose the details of outbreaks of contagious diseases in their territory in order to facilitate the development of vaccines and to prevent the spread of the pandemic? Or, is it the right of state governments to manage the crisis themselves? Case study 1 on p. 71 addresses these issues and the possible tensions between national sovereignty and global health in further detail.

Neoliberalism

Neoliberalism emerges from a broader tradition of liberal thought and the idealist tradition in international relations. Liberal theory is concerned with the individual person rather than collectives. This focus on the well-being of the individual is reflected in the central tenets of neoliberalism. Similarly, the idealist emphasis on the importance and value of international institutions is also retained. However, neoliberalism has also incorporated certain assumptions from the realist school of thought. For example, neoliberals accept the centrality of the state as an actor in IR but, unlike realists, they acknowledge the role and importance of other non-state actors.

Neoliberalism is optimistic about the possibility of collaboration between states in international institutions, although many scholars accept that the institutions are often more effective in facilitating economic and trade relations between states, for example, through the World Trade Organization (WTO), than they are in the field of security. This can be found by examining the problems involved in gaining agreement between the major powers within the United Nations Security Council. Examples of politically contentious issues on which the UN has been unable to act decisively include the crisis in Rwanda in the mid-1990s, or in Dafur in the early 2000s. Perhaps most famously in recent times, the diplomatic stalemate that emerged in the lead-up to the US-led invasion of Iraq in 2003.

Given the concern of liberal theory with the individual, it is unsurprising that neoliberalism focuses on what is termed 'human security' rather than simply state security. Human security focuses on the safety and well-being of individuals within states rather than the security and survival of the states they inhabit. Underpinning this is a belief in fundamental, universal human rights and the doctrine of collective security, which places the responsibility for guaranteeing these rights on the international community, acting under the auspices of international organizations such as the United Nations. For a further discussion on human security, see Chapter 14.

Liberal values, informed by conceptions of a universal right to health, underpin much of the policy agenda in global health. The concept of human security, for example, focuses not only on the threat to individuals from war or oppression by their governments, but has broadened out to include a multitude of other factors such as poverty, disease, and environmental degradation that affect the livelihood and well-being of millions of people across the planet. From a liberal perspective, the HIV and AIDS epidemic, for example, has been considered a (human) security issue and a matter of concern for the international community. For realists, meanwhile, this would be seen as an internal issue for the states in question and the responsibility of those state governments to intervene as they see fit.

In the field of international political economy (IPE), neoliberalism is premised on a belief in the benefits of free trade and the positive effects this can have economically and politically. Economically, states benefit through the greater specialization and the more efficient allocation of resources brought about through international trade, and politically through greater interconnectedness between states as trading partners, which lessens the possibility of conflict between them.

Constructivism

It is necessary to think of constructivism not as a theory but as an overlapping set of related theories or as a general approach to theorizing IR. In the literature, scholars talk about 'thick' and 'thin' or 'strong' and 'weak' versions of the overall approach, which can differ greatly from one another. What underlies constructivist approaches is an emphasis on the need to view events and processes in their (temporal, geographical, cultural, and political) context and to explain them in terms of meaning and identity. Constructivists look to account for the specific historical conditions that led to a given event. They often attempt to trace the emergence of politically salient issues, or the particular terms that structure political debates. This may involve, for example, problematizing and expanding the concept of security or human rights present in global health debates or examining why some issues enter the political agenda while others do not. For example, scholars may focus on how, when, and why HIV/AIDS, malaria, obesity or tobacco control emerged as political issues and how the attempts by certain actors to intervene to tackle these issues were driven forward through a process of political mobilization.

Critical approaches

Like constructivism, critical approaches to IR should be thought of as a collection of associated theories with certain commonalities rather than as a single unified approach to the study of IR. Nevertheless, critical approaches share a common set of aims and objectives. If 'mainstream' approaches look to describe and explain the world, critical approaches look to change it. Most variants of critical theory derive their intellectual inspiration from the works of Karl Marx. Marxist scholars examine the exploitative nature of the international system with the goal of 'emancipation'. Although emancipation is perhaps hard to define in very specific terms, it can be read as an ideal of equality and justice for the entire world's people regardless of nationality or geography and an end to exploitation of the poor by the wealthy and powerful. The Marxist approach within the field of IPE is sometimes termed 'structuralism' in reference to the claim that the existing structures of the global economy are inherently exploitative and must be dismantled and replaced by a fairer system.

Scholars applying critical theory to the study of global health may focus on the unequal access to medicines or clean drinking water for people in certain parts of the world or on the role of economic globalization in preventing this. Equally, a broader question surrounds the connection between health and poverty and the consequences for health of massive economic inequalities between the Global South and the Global North. Some critics have argued that the wealth of Western Europe and North America depends on the exploitation of poverty in their client states elsewhere in the world.

As with other approaches, critical IR theory offers important insights into the global health. Much of the focus in health policy at the national level in recent years has been on structural drivers of health. In the same way, the structural characteristics of the international system, and the economic relations that pertain between states, are key determinants of health in low- and middle-income countries. While some actors focus on issues such as aid and debt relief, critical scholars call for a fundamental reconfiguration of the international economic, trade, and political systems to remove the structural impediments to health in large swathes of the world.

Feminist and post-colonial approaches

While feminist and post-colonial approaches both have overtly Marxist variants – and share the overall goal of emancipation and justice – they must be considered as distinct theoretical traditions. Feminist approaches to IR examine issues of gender in an international context. This may focus on particular conceptions of human security – for example, on the specific experience of women in conflict situations, in which they may be the victims of systematic rape or may face additional dangers and challenges as the primary carers of children. Alternatively, feminist approaches may look more abstractly at the particular forms of male domination, or patriarchy, which structure the conduct and conceptualization of international politics. The relevance of feminist approaches to global health is again obvious, not least in the field of maternal and reproductive health, including contraception and family planning services. In addition, given that women are often the primary carers of children, they are disproportionately impacted by the availability and consequences of specialist paediatric medical services.

Post-colonialism examines issues relating to the developing world as a consequence of colonialism and the position occupied by former colonies and their inhabitants since the process of decolonialization began in the early to mid-twentieth century. Many scholars working within this tradition highlight new forms of colonialism that have emerged within the global economy as a result of the relationship of dependence that exists between former colonies in the developing world and governments and corporations in developed countries. Many of the questions of interest to scholars of global health focus on these types of issues. The burden of disease and poverty falls heavily on those in developing countries whose situation is arguably worsened by the policies of states in the rich world and the global institutions they dominate. In this sense, the focus of post-colonialism is closely related to critical approaches and the structural economic consequences of the post-colonial settlement that exist as a structural determinant of health.

🖉 **Activity 5.2**

Consider which of the above theories offers the most convincing account of international politics. Write one or two paragraphs explaining why you think this is. Use at least one example to support your case.

Feedback

It is argued that realism underplays the ability of international institutions to regulate state behaviour while neoliberalism overstates this. Similarly, some commentators argue that while neoliberal institutionalism provides a sound account in the field of IPE, realism provides the most insightful framework for examining security issues. Constructivists are also open to the challenge that that some interests of states (such as the claim to internal sovereignty over their domestic affairs and their desire for security and survival) are universal and permanent. Post-colonial and feminist approaches meanwhile offer insightful interpretations of particular sets of issues and situations in international relations, but it is claimed they are perhaps unable to provide universal theories of international politics that realists and neoliberals at least claim to be able to provide. Feminist critics may respond to this by saying that they analyse not simply the specific experience of women as a result of certain policies, but the structuring effects of patriarchy on the conduct of international politics. This, it is claimed, is a universal condition structuring all social relations, including the conduct of international relations.

The state and globalization

Processes of globalization have impacted on the state as a political actor both domestically and in the international domain. First, globalization has led to the emergence of new types of global policy and regulatory issues that require global solutions. Examples of these include the regulation of cross-border trade or currency flows, or the health challenges posed by the large-scale movement of people across the globe that may facilitate or accelerate the spread of infectious diseases.

Second, changes in the structure of the global economy have led to an erosion of the political power of states to regulate transnational economic activity. The inability of states to act unilaterally to police the activities of corporations, for example, or to halt the spread of infectious diseases and environmental degradation, undermines their *de facto* control, or sovereignty, over certain policy issues. Questions arise about whether the state is able to respond to the challenges presented by globalization and reassert its control over these issues through new governance structures such as international organizations. At the same time, it has been argued that these forms of governance themselves undermine rather than augment the power of the state. The following section examines in more detail the responses of the state to the challenges posed by globalization. Here we will examine both bilateral and multilateral solutions to the problem of governance in a globalizing world. While multilateral solutions involve the formation of international organizations (e.g. the WHO, the WTO, the UN or the EU) or treaties involving a range of different states, and potentially other non-state actors (e.g. the International Treaty on the Non-Proliferation of Nuclear Weapons), bilateral forms of governance refer to agreements between just two states.

Responses to globalization

International organizations can be seen as a means through which states have attempted to respond to the undermining of their capacity for effective unilateral action and the increasing interdependence between states. International organizations of this type are considered to be multilateral actors as they bring together large numbers of states in a single forum. Examples of such organizations include the United Nations, the World Trade Organization, the World Health Organization, the World Bank and its sister organization the International Monetary Fund, the Organization for Economic Cooperation and Development, the G8, the G20, and the European Union.

A central question in IR that is of great importance for our understanding of global health, is to what extent international organizations (IOs) enhance or undermine the power of the state. On the one hand, states retain a strong input into the decision-making structures of IOs. Whereas other organizations may be officially recognized by IOs or may have observer status, states are full members and are at the heart of the decision-making processes of these organizations. On the other hand, however, not all states have equal political input into these decision-making processes. so some states may retain a high level of control over policies decided within an IO, while smaller, poorer states may have little *de facto* input. Similarly, states do not retain complete control over the organizations they create. The secretariat and officials of international organisations may be able to exert considerable influence over the direction and content of the measures adopted within their institutions. The extent to which they retain control varies between institutions. While most international organizations remain overwhelmingly inter-governmental in nature – depending on the member states for their ultimate authority, and guided in the substance of their position by the most powerful members – other IOs such as the EU have a more robust and influential supranational component in the form of the European Commission. The Commission exercises considerable influence over EU legislation through its right to propose and draft laws that are ratified by the European Parliament and the member states in the body known as the Council.

✏ Activity 5.3

Choose an international organization of interest to you. Using the knowledge of international institutions gained in this chapter, write one or two paragraphs explaining how states are affected by their membership of your chosen organisation. Address the following questions in your answer:

1 In what ways are states able to use these institutions to achieve their aims and objectives?
2 Are some states more able to do this than others?

Feedback

States may be affected in a number of ways by their membership of IOs. International organizations place obligations on states but also confer certain rights. The ability of states to influence these organizations and to pursue their aims and objectives through them will depend on both the formal governance mechanisms of the organization and the *de facto modus operandi*. For example, while the WTO officially works on the basis of one member one vote, in reality, complex trade bargains are the result of power politics. As such, larger, richer states may dictate the terms of the deals struck and the rules enforced.

In addition, the ability of states to enact certain domestic policies may be curtailed by the obligations they have entered into in a certain IO. For example, the Australian Government's decision to introduce plain packaging for tobacco products is being challenged under the WTO law. In theory, if the dispute resolution body finds in favour of the plaintiffs, the Australian Government may have to abandon its policy in order to comply with WTO law.

In addition to the multilateral responses to globalization described above, there are a number of important bilateral relationships that states have entered into both with other states and third-party actors. Bilateral relationships are often associated with the financing of particular health programmes in developing world countries. For example, The President's Emergency Plan for AIDS Relief (PEPFAR), funded by the US Government, established funding for a range of HIV-related programmes in low-income countries. Bilateral programmes serve as a means through which donors can exercise direct control over how its funds are allocated and applied, and also allow funders to promote particular forms of intervention that are in keeping with the underlying ideology of the funder. Elements of the programmes funded by PEPFAR have been criticized on these grounds (Waxman 2004).

Furthermore, bilateral agreements are becoming increasingly common in the field of international trade. As the Doha Round of WTO negotiations stalled in the early 2000, states began to negotiate an increasing number of bilateral and regional trade agreements with one another. These agreements have particular consequences for global health. It has been argued that these agreements prioritize trade over health. For example, they often provide corporations with extensive powers to challenge domestic policies that they feel infringe their economic or intellectual property rights under so-called 'investor state clauses'. These differ from WTO agreements in which only states, not private companies, can bring disputes against other states. Currently, Altria, the owner of Philip Morris tobacco, which is headquartered in Switzerland, is challenging plans by the Uruguay Government to introduce large, graphic warning labels on tobacco products under the Switzerland–Uruguay Bilateral Investment Treaty. Further agreements under negotiation include the Trans-Pacific Partnership (TPP) and the US–EU Free Trade agreement, which will also include investor state measures. Public health actors have argued that a 'carve out' should be made for tobacco from these clauses, meaning they would not apply to this sector, but this has been resisted and, in any case, would not protect other areas of public health policy from different industries. The impact of these trade agreements on health is discussed further in Chapters 8 and 11.

The state and global health governance

Having looked at the effects of globalization on the state in general terms, we turn now to the question of the state as an actor in the field of global health governance. As we have seen, there are particular pressures placed on state actors as a result of globalization. These include not only health issues such as the potentially rapid spread of global pandemics which derive specifically from changes in people's lifestyles brought about as a result of globalization, but issues which have become politicized as a result of the spread of information through mass communications technology. The apparent interconnectedness of the globe and the greater awareness of issues elsewhere in the world have focused the attention of many people in the high-income countries to the health issues faced by those in low- and middle-income countries. Furthermore, there is an increasing awareness of the role that governments and corporations in the developed world have played in either bringing about or maintaining a system of economic and political governance that leads to massive wealth inequalities and the associated consequences for health and well-being. Thus, we can speak about *material* globalization in terms of trade and other forms of interconnection, but also a *psychological* form of globalization that creates an awareness of the problems faced by those thousands of miles away (see the discussions in Chapter 2).

While states may feel compelled to act by the injustice of widespread inequality and adverse public reaction to this at home, they may be unable to respond unilaterally to the health challenges presented by globalization. Instead, these may only be addressable through coordinated, international action. Perhaps as a consequence of this, the past decades have witnessed the emergence of a myriad of non-state actors in the field of global health, including non-governmental organizations (NGOs), charitable organizations, policy networks, and transnational corporations (TNCs). These actors have also acted in concert with states through Global Health Partnerships. These actors and arrangements offer alternative channels of policy delivery and thus challenge the pre-eminence of the state as a global health actor.

Given the emergence of global policy challenges and the range of policy actors outlined above, the question arises of the relative importance of the state versus civil society actors and international organizations. Does the state remain the principal actor in the field of global health? To try and answer this we shall look at case studies of the changing role of the state in two different areas of global health governance. They are introduced here to highlight the role of the state as an actor in each area, but it will be useful for you to cross-reference the issues raised here with the more systematic treatment of these policies elsewhere.

Box 5.1 Case study: The state and the SARS outbreak

The first case study focuses on the 2003 SARS outbreak and the political responses to this as an example of the governance of communicable and infectious diseases more generally. David Fidler (2004) argues that the 2003 outbreak marked the transition from a 'Westphalian' to a 'post-Westphalian' system of governance in the field of communicable diseases. In other words, this marked a transition from a state-centred system based on the sovereignty of states over the treatment of disease outbreaks within their own territory to a system in which the international community, and the international organizations through which it acts, began to play a more robust role in the governance of these issues, intervening in the internal affairs of states in the name of the common welfare of the international community. According to Fidler, the post-Westphalian system is marked by the decentring of the role of the state and the increasing prominence of other, non-state actors. In contrast to Fidler's analysis, James Ricci (2009) argues that the global health governance literature has overstated the extent to which the role of the state in global health governance has diminished or been usurped by other actors, and cites evidence of the continued importance of the state in global health governance.

Box 5.2 Case study: The state and the fight against HIV/AIDS

The crucial issue in the fight against HIV/AIDS centres on access to (very expensive) anti-retroviral medication, or ARVs, by those infected by HIV in developing countries where the majority of the world's known cases of HIV infection are found. Access to these medicines is restricted by the enormous cost of patented drugs and the inability to produce cheaper generic versions of ARVs due to the protection of drug companies' intellectual property rights under international patent law and WTO agreements. Thus there is a conflict between the intellectual property rights of drug companies on the one hand, and the need for drugs by those in the developing world on the other.

State actors have played a crucial role in bringing about the current state of affairs. It was state actors who concluded the Uruguay Round of negotiations that brought the WTO into being, along with the agreement, Trade Related Aspects of Intellectual Property (TRIPS), which is designed to protect intellectual property rights. In particular, the US Government was vital in negotiating the TRIPS agreement at the WTO and insisted on the inclusion of protection for pharmaceuticals in it.

In addition, states also provide the 'hardware' of public health care (Fidler 2007). They often produce the overall strategies for tackling health issues like HIV/AIDS and state agencies play a central role in implementing these strategies on the ground (Wogart et al. 2009). The governments of high-income countries provide overseas aid that is used to tackle issues such as HIV/AIDS through agencies such USAID, the US International Development Agency, or the Department for International Development (DFID) in the UK.

There are various *supranational bodies* and IOs active in the field of HIV/AIDS, including the World Bank Multi-country AIDS Projects, the G8, the Office of the United Nations High Commissioner for Refugees (UNHCR). and UNAIDS; however, it is crucial to remember that states play a vital role in the governance and funding of IOs. In addition to state and supranational bodies, there are *global health partnerships*, most notably the Global Fund to Fight AIDS, Tuberculosis and Malaria ('the Global Fund), which involves a variety of different agencies and actors working together. It should also be noted that although these actors play an important role in the fight against AIDS, it is states that provide the overwhelming majority of funding channelled through the Global Fund.

Together with the Global Fund, *civil society organizations* (CSOs) have played a crucial role in bringing the issue of ARVs onto the agenda. CSOs such as Médecins Sans Frontières and the Red Cross are also involved in the treatment of patients and the distribution of medication in many developing countries. The process of tackling HIV/AIDS thus involves a complex interplay of state and non-state actors and it is difficult to assess the relative contribution made by these actors to that fight.

✏️ **Activity 5.4**

Think about the areas of global health governance we have looked at. In which areas has the state played the most important role? In which areas has its role been usurped by other actors? Which actors were these and why did they assume the role they did? Summarize your findings in a brief paragraph giving examples to support your points.

Re-read the definition of the state you wrote at the start of the chapter. Reflect on whether your understanding of the state has changed and, if so, how. If your understanding has changed, write a new definition of the role of the state that reflects your current understanding.

Summary

In summary, we have seen that the state continues to be a vitally important actor in domestic and international politics. There are various theoretical approaches to understanding its very different roles in each of these domains. There are also an increasing number of non-state actors that are of varying importance in different areas of global health governance. Nevertheless, states arguably remain the most important of all of these actors, playing a vital role in all areas of public health policy both directly and through the international organizations they govern and fund.

References

Dahl, R.A. (1961) *Who Governs? Power and Democracy in an American City*. New Haven, CT: Yale University Press.

Fidler, D.P. (2004) *SARS: Governance and the Globalization of Disease*. London: Palgrave Macmillan.

Fidler, D. (2007) Architecture amidst anarchy: global health's quest for governance, *Global Health Governance*, 1 (1) [www.ghgj.org/Fidler_Architecture.pdf].

Hobbes, T. (1960) *Leviathan: Or the Matter, Forme and Power of a Commonwealth Ecclesiasticall and Civil*. New Haven, CT: Yale University Press.

Locke, J. (1988) *Locke: Two Treatises of Government* (student edn). Cambridge: Cambridge University Press.

Miliband, R. (1969) *The State in Capitalist Society*. London: Weidenfeld & Nicolson.

Ricci, J. (2009) Global health governance and the state: premature claims of a post-international framework, *Global Health*, III (1): 1–18.

Skocpol, T. (1979) *States and Social Revolutions*. Cambridge: Cambridge University Press.

Waxman, H.A. (2004). Politics of international health in the Bush Administration, *Development*, 47 (2): 24–8.

Weber, M. (1972) *Politics as a Vocation*. Philadelphia, PA: Fortress Press.

Wogart, J.P., Calcagnotto, G., Hein, W. and van Soest, C. (2009) AIDS and access to medicines: Brazil, South Africa and global health governance, in K. Buse, W. Hein and N. Drager (eds) *Making Sense of Global Health Governance: A Policy Perspective*. Basingstoke: Palgrave Macmillan.

Commercial actors and global health governance

6

Benjamin Hawkins

Overview

In this chapter, you will learn about the involvement of the commercial sector in global health governance. Commercial actors, such as transnational corporations, are increasingly important actors in global health. Thus any account of the field of global health governance (GHG) that ignores corporate actors is incomplete. Here we address the role played by commercial actors in GHG and explore their motivation for participating in different types of governance arrangement.

Learning objectives

After working through this chapter, you will be able to:

- define the commercial sector and differentiate it from other global health actors
- assess the changing role of corporations and the nature of corporate power in the context of globalization
- evaluate the roles played by transnational corporations in global health governance
- critically assess the motivation behind companies' corporate social responsibility programmes

Key terms

Corporate social responsibility: Industry-supported measures whereby companies attempt to demonstrate responsible behaviour.

Corporation: An association of stockholders that is regarded as an artificial person under most national laws. Ownership is marked by ease of transferability and stockholders have limited liability.

Intellectual property: Creations of the mind, including inventions, literary and artistic works, and symbols, names, images and designs. It is of two types: industrial (e.g. patents and trademarks) and copyright (e.g. music and films).

Regulation: The enforcement of norms, standards, rules, and principles that govern behaviour.

Regulatory capture: An economic term describing a situation where a market actor uses its power, resources, and influence to obtain regulatory outcomes that advance its interests.

Defining the commercial sector

When we talk about the commercial sector, we are referring to private actors, such as corporations that exist explicitly to produce profits. As set out in Chapter 3, in the context of global health policy, we often focus on transnational corporations, active in multiple countries. However, the commercial sector includes organizations that are not-for-profit in their legal status, registered, for example, with charitable status, but which are established to support a particular firm or industry. These may include business federations, such as the International Federation of Pharmaceutical Manufacturers Associations (IFPMA). Similarly, not-for-profit organizations established by companies or wealthy individuals but run at an arm's length from them (e.g. the Soros Foundation) are included here as many foundations have injected both large quantities of resources and commercial mindset into the global health sector. A list of different types of organizations which fall within the corporate sector is set out in Box 6.1.

Box 6.1 Types of commercial sector organization

- Business associations, established to promote their members' interests, such as the International Chamber of Commerce (ICC).
- Associations of privately employed professionals with an interest in global health, such as the International Private Practitioners Association.
- Non-profit, issue-specific, industry-funded think-tanks, and institutes with interests in global health. For example, documents from the tobacco company Philip Morris reveal that it provided US$880,000 to create the Institute of Regulatory Policy in the USA 'as a vehicle [to lobby] for the executive order on risk assessment', aiming to delay the publication of an EPA report on environmental tobacco smoke (Muggli et al. 2004).
- Non-profit 'patient groups' established to advance industry interests. For example, the International Alliance of Patients' Organizations is registered as a charitable foundation in the Netherlands and funded by Pharmaceutical Partners for Better Healthcare, a consortium of about 30 major companies. It has over 100 member patient organizations and a stated interest in improving patient voice. Its hidden agenda is likely to support consumer advertising and public/insurance funding of specific treatments.
- Industry front organizations, including non-profit, industry-established and industry-funded scientific organizations with an interest in health issues. For example, the International Life Sciences Institute supports industry-friendly science and attempts to influence regulation in areas such as diet, tobacco, and alcohol.
- Non-profit, philanthropic organizations that invest resources in global health, influence global priorities and approaches, and leverage additional commercial sector involvement (e.g. the Bill and Melinda Gates Foundation).
- Loose, issue-oriented networks. ARISE (Associates for Research into the Science of Enjoyment) publishes articles promoting the pleasures of 'smoking, alcohol, caffeine and chocolate', and receives funding from companies such as Coca-Cola, Miller Beer, and Kraft.
- Virtual service providers (e.g. World Directory of Holistic Practitioners), virtual communities, and virtual campaigners. Internet sites can also serve as fronts for commercial organizations.

The defining feature of the commercial sector is its market orientation and the pursuit of profit. Thus, while corporations may have additional societal, environmental or other objectives, these are necessarily secondary to the underlying search for profit. A further defining feature of corporations is that they have a particular legal status independent of their ownership. They have the status of a 'legal person', allowing corporations to enjoy specific rights and legal protections. Corporations' attempts to protect their rights – for example, the intellectual property rights of pharmaceutical companies – are at the centre of many current debates in global health governance.

🖉 Activity 6.1

Select a global health issue with which you are familiar and list the commercial organizations relevant to it. Identify one or two examples for each of the types of organization listed in Table 6.1. Complete the table by listing the interests of these organizations in the issue, the roles that they play in relation to the issue, and their impact on health.

Table 6.1 Commercial organizations active in a selected global health issue

Type of organization	Name of organizations	Interests in the issue	Roles in the issue	Impact on health
Transnational corporations	1. 2.			
Business associations	1. 2.			
Professional associations	1. 2.			
Standards organizations	1. 2.			
Think-tanks	1. 2.			
Patient groups	1. 2.			
Scientific networks	1. 2.			
Philanthropic organizations	1 2.			
Loose networks	1. 2.			
Tight networks	1. 2.			
Virtual organizations	1. 2.			

Feedback

It should be clear by now that although the commercial sector comprises those organizations established to realize a profit for their owners, consideration of the sector's role in global health also requires recognition of those organizations that may be non-profit but serve corporate ends. By adopting this approach, a vast range of commercially oriented organizations and networks with an interest in global health emerge. The sector is highly differentiated with organizations varying by size, kinds of resources (financial capital, technology, employment, and natural resources), level of formalization, geographical scope, compliance with the rule of law, as well as by their interest in global health governance.

Commercial interests in global governance

The increasing movement of goods, services, people, and capital between states that has occurred as a result of globalization has created the need for global rules and regulatory regimes that are able to govern these process and the organizations at their heart. Consequently, the period since the Second World War has seen the emergence of a variety of international organizations, including the World Health Organization, the World Bank, and the World Trade Organization.

The emergence of a global economy has been characterized by tremendous growth in the number and scale of global firms. While globalization presents new opportunities for profit, it also presents challenges to these global companies. As firms expand their reach, they have an increasing need for rules to govern their transactions on a global basis. Such rules serve to minimize uncertainty and lower transaction costs associated with information gathering, negotiation, and enforcement. International regimes and global regulations have certain advantages for transnational corporations. They minimize uncertainty, create common standards allowing the production of uniform products, and reduce transaction costs. However, as with corporations in the domestic sphere, transnational corporations have a preference for self-regulation and for establishing their own codes of practice over government-mandated regulations.

Activity 6.2

Make a list of reasons why health policy-makers should pay attention to the role(s) of the commercial sector in global health governance. In framing your response, consider the nature of global health problems, the capacity of the state to address them, and the assets of the commercial sector.

Feedback

Your answer might include any of the following considerations. Health impacts of trans-border flows often exceed the regulatory capacity of governments, whether acting alone or collectively through inter-governmental organizations. These include the illicit trade of goods and services (and persons), the spread of antimicrobial resistance and pathogens, emerging and re-emerging infectious diseases, environmental pollution, information and communication, and population migration. Since the commercial sector often plays a key role in the flow of people and things across borders (along with other actors), we need to rethink classical state-centric public health approaches to dealing with them. How should the commercial sector be involved in governing the consequences of cross-border flows in ways that can contribute to public health goals? In addition, corporations' economic power and their role as political actors in global health governance make them impossible to ignore.

Corporations and the provision of health care

Corporations may be the direct providers of many core health services, such as residential care homes for the elderly, optometry practices, and private hospitals. As well as services, they produce a range of goods required to diagnose and treat illnesses, such as scanning machines and medications. Increasingly, health services as well as health care equipment are being traded across borders. In many countries, corporations are providers of health insurance and are involved in the financing and construction of the health service infrastructure. Finally, corporations play a significant role in the health and well-being of those they employ by providing safe working environments and support for employees suffering from physical and mental illnesses.

Corporations and the production of ill health

The activities of transnational corporations producing tobacco, alcoholic beverages, and foods high in sugar, salt, and fat are associated with a number of chronic diseases, which are now the principal causes of death in developed countries. Increasingly, they are also impacting developing countries.

Economic significance

In addition to the involvement of corporations in both the production and treatment of ill health, their economic strength means they are simply too large and important a group of actors to ignore. Indeed, their economic resources often dwarf those of international organizations and even states. When seen in these terms, the potential impact of corporations on global health is clear. The economic strength of transnational corporations means they wield formidable political strength. There is clear evidence that corporations attempt to influence the policy process to defend their business interests and that they enjoy a high degree of success in gaining this influence (Holden and Lee 2009). In order to influence policy, corporations target government at the local, national, and supranational levels.

Corporations as political actors

The aim of corporations in the political sphere can be summarized by the term *regulatory capture*. This is defined as a situation where a market actor uses its power, resources, and/or influence to obtain regulatory outcomes that advance its interests. This often involves corporations advancing the narrow commercial interest of that organization over broader public interest. It is facilitated by regulatory bodies systematically favouring the interests of corporations over those of the citizens they govern. Transnational corporations with an interest in, or impact on, health will almost invariably be engaged in the direct lobbying of governments directly and through public affairs consultancies whose services they retain for this specific purpose.

In addition, there are a number of other channels available to corporations, through which they are able to engage with, and potentially influence, the policy process. Many of the actors set out in Box 6.1 play important roles in this context.

Analysing corporate power

It is useful to think of corporate power in terms of structure and agency (Farnsworth and Holden 2006). Structural power is derived from the privileged position capital owners occupy in the market economy. Agency power is based on direct social relations and refers to the deliberate exercise of influence.

Structural power

Structural power is based on control over investment. A state may be dependent on the revenue generated by the activities of a corporation, the foreign direct investment it provides, and/or the employment it creates. An obvious example of this is the duty paid on cigarettes or alcohol, which have proved major barriers towards effective regulation of these industries as finance ministries fear the loss of revenue from lower levels of consumption of these products. Similarly, governments may be sympathetic to the case of pharmaceutical companies who provide employment, corporation tax revenues, and, not least, life-saving medicines.

Many scholars have argued that the structural power of corporations has increased in the context of globalization, because it has provided transnational corporations with the 'capacity for exit'. In other words, they are able to relocate from one country to another to seek more favourable conditions (e.g. the tax regime). The effect of relocation is a loss of corporation tax revenue and potentially even more wide-reaching effects in terms of economic growth, employment, public spending, and welfare costs. In countries where the government is reliant on a single industry or even a single corporation for the majority of its income, the threat of exit is a powerful tool.

Corporations also have ideological influence over governments and citizens. Within much of the world, and particularly in the developed world, there is a high level of acceptance for the pro-business ideas popularized by corporate actors favouring free markets, deregulation, and low levels of taxation. Business leaders are venerated and the private sector is revered as the engine of economic growth. Indeed, many of these ideas are treated as unquestionable truths in certain sections of the media and there is no shortage of willing mouthpieces for the pro-business message. This is unsurprising since private-sector actors, including some of the world's largest and most powerful corporations (e.g. News Corporation; see Chapter 1), control much of the media. The result of this is that it is seen as acceptable for corporations to be present in ever-expanding areas of public life, including in the development and implementation of public policy.

Agency power

Agency power may take the form of political engagement, such as lobbying governments, regulatory bodies, and international organizations (IOs), or through related activities such as the funding of political parties or campaigns for office. However, there are more subtle, less obvious processes through which corporations act to further their interests. One way of doing this is participation in various institutions and agencies involved in the formulation or delivery of policy, such as occupying seats on management boards of service providers. In addition, corporations may be involved in government committees or state delegations to international organizations. In this way, the attempts by corporations to influence the policy process may focus on all levels of that process: local, national, regional (for example, the EU), and even global. Their presence in these forums is in large part the result of their attempts to depict themselves as 'stakeholders' in the policy process, with particular expertise in a certain sector which enables them to contribute to the formulation of good policies and the ability to oversee their effective implementation on the ground.

Expertise

The expertise possessed by corporations is a crucial resource of power. It is often invaluable to policy-makers supporting corporations' claims to be key stakeholders in the policy process. Corporations are often the main (or even only) source of cutting-edge technical expertise in a given area. At times, corporations will also produce evidence to support their aims and objectives through sponsorship of scientists or scientific institutes sympathetic to their cause.

Three approaches to global health governance

There are three principal ways in which corporations seek to influence global health governance: influencing public regulation, co-regulation, and self-regulation by private standards. Where possible, business seeks to establish its own rules through self-regulation and co-regulatory regimes. Where this is not possible, it seeks to influence public regulation through international organizations such as the World Trade Organization and the United Nations. Let us now examine each of these forms of engagement in global health governance in turn.

Influencing public regulation

Corporations can exert influence at each of the stages of the policy process set out here. They will look to use all available channels through which they can engage either the officials involved in the drafting of legislation or parliamentarians who will enact it into law. Equally, once laws are in place, there is often substantial debate about the way in which they are to be implemented and enforced and how their impacts are to be evaluated, which industry actors can seek to influence. A range of corporate influencing tactics are set out in Box 6.2.

Box 6.2 Corporate influencing strategies

- Delaying the introduction of international instruments (e.g. conventions, codes, agreements). For example, it is alleged that during the 1980s, the IFPMA delayed WHO efforts on a code of pharmaceutical marketing by arguing that it required time to implement its own voluntary code (Richter 2001).
- Blocking the adoption of an instrument. For example, the sugar industry provided the main opposition to the international dietary guidelines proposed by the WHO in 2003.
- Influencing the content of an instrument. For example, tobacco companies lobbied at the national and international levels to secure changes to the text of the Framework Convention on Tobacco Control.
- Challenging the credibility/validity of the instruments. For example, the global alcohol industry represented by bodies such as the Scotch Whisky Association has repeatedly challenged the internationally accepted evidence base on the effectiveness of minimum unit pricing to reduce alcohol-related harm (McCambridge et al. 2013).
- Undermining the legitimacy and capacity of an international organization charged with negotiating an instrument. An enquiry into the influence of the tobacco industry in WHO revealed that an elaborate, well-financed, sophisticated, and usually invisible global effort had been undertaken by the industry 'to divert attention from public health issues, to reduce budgets for the scientific and policy activities carried out by WHO, to pit other UN agencies against WHO, to convince developing countries that WHO's tobacco control programme was a "first world" agenda carried out at the expense of the developing world, to distort the results of important scientific studies, and to discredit WHO as an institution' (Zeltner et al. 2000).
- Challenging the competence of a UN body to develop norms in a particular domain. For example, the food industry has tried to circumscribe the extent to which WHO can address obesity by proposing policies and regulations (Waxman 2004).
- Using legal challenges under international trade agreements to stymie public health regulations. The global tobacco industry has used WTO agreements and Bilateral Investment Treaties (e.g. between Hong Kong and Australia) to challenge the introduction of generic packaging for cigarettes.

A great deal of effort is spent on agenda formulation, which may mean pushing issues of importance on to the political agenda by lobbying officials or elected politicians or by trying to influence broader societal debates through the media. Equally, corporations may be keen to keep certain issues off the agenda and may employ a similar range of tactics to do this and to divert attention onto other issues that are either beneficial to them or are not considered to pose the same level of threat. At the legislative phase, corporations may be invited to provide evidence to public enquiries or to appear as witnesses to parliamentary committees, or may seek out opportunities to do so.

A further tactic available to corporations is to propose or initiate measures that advance corporate interests, or which promote ineffective regulations that will not impede their core business activities. Equally, they will seek to delay or ideally block the adoption of a policy or instrument that runs counter to their interests, or to frustrate the implementation of that policy if adopted. This may involve a variety of activities, including questioning the effectiveness of a policy or the evidence base on which it depends, or drawing attention to the supposed negative side-effects of its implementation in order to call for caution and restraint in legislation.

In addition to the overtures made to governments and policy-makers, corporations may use a variety of media to influence public perceptions of the effectiveness of a particular policy instrument in order to marshal opposition against it and reduce the likelihood of governments (in democratic states at least) pursuing the measures in question.

Box 6.3 Case study: The TRIPs agreement

The creation of the World Trade Organization (WTO) and the agreement on Trade Related Aspects of Intellectual Property Rights (TRIPS) introduced intellectual property law into the international trading system for the first time.

A crucial role was played by US corporations in influencing the negotiating position of the US delegation during the Uruguay Round and thus, given the huge political sway that the US holds over the content of international trade agreements, the content of the WTO agreement itself. The corporations in question were able to engage with the negotiation process at each of the stages highlighted above, helping to set the agenda for negotiations, participating in and influencing the negotiations of the agreement itself and the subsequent application and enforcement of that agreement.

Setting the agenda on TRIPs
In 1986, the CEOs of twelve US-based corporations formed a body called the Intellectual Property Committee, or IPC, the purpose of which was to seek a comprehensive agreement on intellectual property within the context of the Uruguay Round of negotiations which created the WTO. The IPC acted as a coordinating body for the lobbying activities of the most powerful corporations in America as they attempted to influence the US Government's negotiating position. This involved initially getting intellectual property on to the radar of US trade delegations and ensuring that it would have a prominent place in the Uruguay Round of negotiations.

Drafting TRIPS
The IPC hired a trade lawyer, Jaques Gorlin, to draft an international intellectual property treaty that would secure these interests. The resultant draft was adopted by the US administration as the basis of its negotiating position. In addition, the CEO of Pfizer, a leading pharmaceutical producer, acted as an advisor to the US delegation during the Uruguay negotiations. Given the support of the US Government, the IPC was successful in translating its interests into law and seeing its draft treaty form the basis of the TRIPS agreement. According to Gorlin, the agreement almost entirely reflects the corporations' agenda, with the IPC getting '95% of what it wanted' included in the final text of the agreement (Sell 2003).

This alignment of the government of the most powerful state in the world with the most powerful corporations in the world is noteworthy, as it symbolized an important blurring of the lines between the state and the private sector and raises questions about whose interests the US delegation was representing in the negotiations: those of the powerful corporate elite or the American people more generally? TRIPS marks a new departure in the role of corporate actors in the political sphere, not simply in terms of the strategy adopted by corporations and the political influence they were able to gain over governments, but the international dimension of these ramifications. As Sell (2003: 96) comments: 'In effect, twelve corporations made public law for the world.'

Governance implications of TRIPS

While TRIPS represents a shift in authority from the state to the private sector, it did not mean that corporations have completely usurped the authority of the state or that states could be bypassed altogether. The TRIPS negotiations demonstrate the continued importance of the state in the international sphere and its role in negotiating and concluding international agreements. Equally, it is states that enact and enforce intellectual property laws in the domestic sphere. Nevertheless, TRIPS demonstrated the blurring of the lines between governments and the private sector and the extent to which corporations are able to influence the negotiating positions of the former. Corporate influence in this sector has arguably been extended by the inclusion of investor state clauses in regional and bilateral trade agreements concluded after TRIPs.

Co-regulation

In other areas of policy the approach by corporate actors differs. Their aims and objectives may not be to influence the content of particular laws or policies, but to position themselves as partners in the delivery of certain policy measures. This amounts to a deal between public authorities and private sector organizations, often involving civil society as well as corporate actors. While examples of co-regulator regimes are common at the national level, the most obvious example of this type of governance structure at the global level is the UN Global Compact (see following case study).

Co-regulation presents a third way between traditional public, statutory regulation and private self-regulation. It has arisen due to the inadequacies of public and private regulation. The former, it has been argued, is inadequate in an era of globalization as state and inter-governmental capacity for regulation lags behind technological advances made by industry. Furthermore, it can be difficult for national governments to enforce national regimes unilaterally and global regulatory regimes are difficult to achieve and even harder to enforce. Nonetheless, private self-regulation is not always in the public's interest and thus a case remains for some external public control or hook on self-regulation. Co-regulation can be seen as public sector involvement in business self-regulation.

The idea is that the public and private sector negotiate on an agreed set of policy or regulatory objectives that are results-oriented. Subsequently, the private sector takes responsibility for implementation of the provisions. Monitoring compliance may remain a public responsibility or otherwise be contracted out to a third party – sometimes an interested non-governmental organization. The advent of co-regulation is relatively new, and there has been more formal experimentation with it at the national and regional levels. The European Union, for example, is experimenting with co-regulation particularly with respect to the Internet, journalism, and e-commerce. The UN's Global Compact with industry might be viewed as a form of co-regulation, together with many of the global public–private partnerships (PPPs).

Box 6.4 Case study: The UN Global Compact

The UN Global Compact is the first attempt to regulate the activities of transnational corporations at the global level via the UN. It set out a number of principles to guide the conduct of corporations and ensure they act in compliance with a set of ethical standards relating to human rights, labour standards, environmental protection, and the fight against corruption. These include commitments to do the following:

- support and respect the protection of internationally proclaimed human rights;
- ensure they are not complicit in human rights abuses;
- uphold the freedom of association and the effective recognition of the right to collective bargaining;
- eliminate all forms of forced and compulsory labour;
- abolish child labour;
- eliminate discrimination in employment;
- support a precautionary approach to environmental challenges;
- undertake initiatives to promote greater environmental responsibility;
- encourage the development and diffusion of environmentally friendly technologies;
- ensure businesses work against all forms of corruption, including extortion and bribery.

The Compact has been criticized for being voluntary and largely unenforceable, while offering the mark of respectability to companies. These include corporations active in controversial industries, such as the oil and tobacco industries, although in the case of British American Tobacco, their overtures have to date been rebuffed.

In addition, the Compact has been criticized as undermining more robust forms of regulation. While the hope of the UN was to 'fill a void between regulatory regimes, at one end of the spectrum, and voluntary codes of industry, at the other' (Global Compact Office, 2002: 4), in practice, the Compact reinforces 'the pendulum swing away from stricter forms of regulation' (Utting 2002).

Self-regulation

In addition to influencing policy and co-regulation, many corporations advocate the advantages of self-regulation over government legislation or compulsorily regulations. There are two principal types of self-regulation: regulating 'market standards' and 'social standards', respectively. In practice, however, it can be difficult to distinguish between self-regulation of market and social standards, as some mechanisms pursue both goals. In the case of market standards, products, process, and business practice may be subject to governance to support commerce (e.g. to reduce transaction costs or increase confidence in a product). Although such self-regulation may have social impacts, the overriding purpose of market standards is to enable commerce.

By contrast, self-regulation through social standards involves business and industry voluntarily adopting and observing specific practices based on public or social concern rather than to improve the functioning of the market. Self-regulatory social standards are usually developed in response to consumer concerns or boycotts, shareholder activism, or the threat of impending public regulation. Self-regulation of social standards occurs through mechanisms including voluntary codes and reporting initiatives, statements of principles, guidelines and codes of practice, and some public–private partnerships as well as corporate social responsibility activities (discussed below). Self-regulatory initiatives often address issues that are already subject to (often ineffective) statutory regulation. For example, the International Labour Organization (ILO) has issued standards governing maternity leave and breastfeeding at work; some countries have adopted the standards (e.g. India), others have not (e.g. Kenya), while implementation is often partial.

It has been argued that voluntary codes can bring new stakeholders into the regulatory process. For example, temporary labourers, often women, have participated in developing workplace codes, having not typically been represented in comparable ILO processes.

Second, codes may generate better compliance than public regulation. Experience with many international conventions governing social and economic issues suggests that ratifying governments often fail to implement them, but cannot be held accountable by the international community for such failure. In theory, companies adopt codes to gain market share and comply with them to retain the confidence of their consumers/share-holders. Third, codes are less costly to the public sector than statutory regulation.

There are many reasons for scepticism regarding the ability of voluntary codes to adequately govern many global health issues. One review of a large number of codes concludes that codes typically comprise lofty statements of intent, are largely responsive to consumer pressure, and highlight issues in consumer-sensitive industries (e.g. apparel) while ignoring many others. Moreover, companies generally lack the means to communicate compliance in reliable and believable ways. Codes have been further criticized because of their emphasis on company 'commitment' rather than holding companies legally accountable to ensuring specific rights. Consequently, such patchwork self-regulation may result in 'enclave' social policy, governing select issues and groups of workers at specific points in their working lives. Such self-regulatory efforts may erode societal commitment to universal rights and entitlements in the process.

Since codes of practice are voluntary, they are not traceable to public authority. Consequently, they are open to the same criticisms in terms of accountability as co-regulatory regimes. Issues arise in terms of enforcement, which is undertaken by market actors themselves rather than by an external or government agency. This has led self-regulatory regimes to be criticized as toothless and unable to force measures upon corporations unwilling to comply. This is especially the case when dealing with the largest and most powerful corporations. Finally, these regimes are criticized in terms of transparency. Since they are instituted and governed by the same corporate actors they are designed to regulate, they are not subject to public monitoring or oversight. The internal workings of self-regulatory regimes often remain opaque to those outside the industry itself, and there are few mechanisms by which these regimes can be called to account.

✎ Activity 6.3

Why might a company commit itself to adhering to a voluntary code? Suggest four to five reasons.

Feedback

While serving social purposes, codes can serve important business functions and ultimately increase profits. Your answer should also include some of the following reasons why codes may improve profitability:

- to demonstrate responsiveness to societal concerns;
- to provide material for public relations;
- to differentiate itself from competitors to increase sales;
- to respond to concerns of consumers to increase sales;
- to respond to concerns of shareholders and encourage greater investment;
- to decrease costs. The British mining conglomerate, Anglo American PLC, estimates that 30,000 of its employees in South Africa are infected with HIV. It has

voluntarily adopted a code in relation to treatment of 3000 employees, costs being
reportedly offset by sharp declines in mortality and absenteeism due to illness.
- to stave off or delay statutory regulation. The tobacco, pharmaceutical, and food
  safety codes mentioned above were advanced to pre-empt more onerous international obligations.
- to provide flexible tools tailored to specific problems instead of blanket regulations
  covering all contingencies.

Corporate social responsibility

Corporate social responsibility (CSR) is a loose umbrella term incorporating a diverse set
of measures undertaken by companies to improve the impact their activities have on the
social environments in which they are present. A more cynical interpretation of CSR may
conclude that its main objective is not to change corporate behaviour or the impacts of
this, but to change the perception of that behaviour among governments and the general
public. In the case of the former, CSR may be seen as an attempt to ward off further
regulation of the industry or to buttress existing self-regulatory regimes that are favourable to the business. In the case of the latter, CSR may work to improve the image of a
corporation in the minds of consumers, to set it aside from competitors, and to win customers on the basis of its ethical or responsible business policies. There has been a rapid
expansion of interest in CSR in recent years in response to a huge increase in corporate
focus in this area. This in turn may be seen as a response to increased concern about
environmental sustainability and the social impact of corporate activity among consumers
and mounting criticism of some corporate behaviour.

In broad terms, CSR may be considered as a strategy that might serve three types of
company:

- Those with social and environmental principles genuinely at the core of their business;
  examples of this type of company include Fairtrade, Body Shop, and the Cooperative
  Bank, which place a great emphasis on their ethical lending policies.
- Corporations aiming to create a link between their brand and social responsibility programmes via partnerships and joint marketing activities. An example here is the public
  relations campaign of clothes maker Benetton and its connection to the World Food
  Programme.
- Controversial industries that are responding to pressure from consumers, investors or
  regulators. An obvious example here is the tobacco industry, which has been the subject
  of extensive regulation over the last few decades and has received considerable criticism
  for its marketing strategies and its attempts to cover up the health risks associated with
  cigarette smoke through a variety of underhand measures.

There is evidence that tobacco corporations saw CSR measures focusing on environmental protection and the eradication of child labour in the field of tobacco cultivation as being
important ways through which they are able to repair their image and fend off calls for still
further regulation of their markets (Fooks et al. 2011).

Summary

In summary, we have seen that corporations are incredibly powerful economic and political actors that play an active role in almost every aspect of global health policy. There is a wide range of mechanisms open to corporations and an equally wide range of tactics they employ to influence policy. In recent decades, their influence has increased in line with underlying ideological shifts in society and an increasingly firm commitment to neoliberal ideas about the effectiveness of markets and private sector actors in delivering social goods. However, the move towards co-regulation and self-regulation, which this ideological shift has ushered in, raises a number of issues about accountability and effectiveness. Should corporations be involved in setting the rules that govern them and what are the consequences of this for global health? These issues are explored further in the following chapter, which includes discussions on global public partnerships and the influence of philanthropic foundations.

References

Farnsworth, K. and Holden, C. (2006) The business–social policy nexus: corporate power and corporate inputs into social policy, *Journal of Social Policy*, 35 (3): 473–94.

Fooks, G.J., Gilmore, A.B., Smith, K.E., Collin, J., Holden, C. and Lee, K. (2011) Corporate social responsibility and access to policy élites: an analysis of tobacco industry documents, *PLoS Medicine*, 8 (8): e1001076.

Global Compact Office (2002) *The Global Compact: Report on Progress and Activities*. New York: United Nations.

Holden, C. and Lee, K. (2009) Corporate power and social policy: the political economy of the transnational tobacco companies, *Global Social Policy*, 9 (3): 328–54.

McCambridge, J., Hawkins, B. and Holden, C. (2013) Industry use of evidence to influence alcohol policy: a case study of submissions to the 2008 Scottish government consultation, *PLoS Medicine*, 10 (4): e1001431.

Muggli, M.E., Hurt, R.D. and Repace, J. (2004) The tobacco industry's political efforts to derail the EPA report on ETS, *American Journal of Preventive Medicine*, 26 (2): 167–77.

Richter, J. (2001) *Holding Corporations Accountable: Corporate Conduct, International Codes, and Citizen Action*. Basingstoke: Palgrave Macmillan.

Sell, S.K. (2003) *Private Power, Public Law: The Globalization of Intellectual Property Rights*. Cambridge: Cambridge University Press.

Utting, P. (2002) The Global Compact and civil society: averting a collision course, *Development in Practice*, 12 (5): 644–7.

Waxman, H.A. (2004) Politics of international health in the Bush Administration, *Development*, 47 (2): 24–8.

Zeltner, T., Kessler, D., Martiny, A. and Randera, F. (2000) *Tobacco Company Strategies to Undermine Tobacco Control Activities at the World Health Organization*. Geneva: World Health Organization.

Non-government actors in global health

7

Neil Spicer

Overview

In this chapter, we look at three 'new' types of global health actor: global civil society organizations, philanthropic foundations, and global health initiatives and partnerships. Each type of actor is described and defined and we look at some of their roles and ways they seek to influence global health issues. We then consider some of the important challenges they have brought to global health governance.

Learning objectives

After working through this chapter, you will be able to:

- understand what is meant by the terms global civil society, philanthropic foundations, and global health partnerships and initiatives
- describe the roles and assess the increasing significance to global health governance of these actors
- consider key opportunities and challenges to global health governance stemming from these actors

Key terms

Global civil society: Organizations, institutions, networks, individuals, ideas, and values located between family, state, and market and operating beyond national societies, policies, and economies.

Global health partnerships and initiatives: Entities for coordinating and financing programmes for specific health problems or diseases, research and development, donating drugs, vaccines or other products, strengthening health systems, campaigning and advocacy, technical assistance or health service and system support.

Philanthropic foundations: Non-profit, non-governmental actors possessing a fund of their own, managed by trustees and directors, and promoting public welfare that includes social, educational, charitable, religious or other activities.

Emerging (new) actors in global health

Shifts in global health governance have brought opportunities and challenges. Substantial increases in development assistance for health, from US$5 billion in 1990 to US$21.8

billion in 2007 (IHME 2009), have occurred in parallel with a growth – some would say a proliferation – of global health actors. As Dodd et al. (2007) explain: 'There are now well over a 100 major international organizations involved in health, far more than in any other sector, and literally hundreds of channels for delivering health aid.'

New types of global health actors are emerging, and the importance of different actors is changing. 'Traditional' actors, namely the bilateral donors and health-related multilaterals such as the World Health Organization, UNICEF, and the World Bank, remain important and influential in global health. 'New' actors, such as philanthropic foundations and other civil society organizations, and global health initiatives and partnerships, are emerging as increasingly significant at the global level (Walt et al. 2009). Such actors have been welcomed for the new resources they can harness and the flexibility and creative thinking they can bring to bear in tackling persistent and emerging global health problems, such as HIV/AIDS. However, they have also exaggerated existing, and indeed introduced a number of new, challenges to global health governance that we will look at later in this chapter.

Global civil society organizations

Civil society can be defined as: 'associations of citizens (outside their families, friends and businesses) entered into voluntarily to advance their interests, ideas and ideologies. The term does not include profit-making activity (the private sector) or governing (the public sector)' (UN 2004). This seemingly straightforward definition obscures a considerable diversity of organizations, including: labour unions, faith-based groups, professional associations, academic and research institutions, think-tanks, human rights networks, consumer rights coalitions, social movements, social and sports clubs, philanthropic foundations, clubs, and indeed criminal organizations and networks (Rowson 2005). When we talk about civil society organizations (CSOs), we usually mean 'public interest' CSOs that aim to benefit the public whether as a whole or particular groups, often but not necessarily vulnerable or marginalized communities. But 'private interest' CSOs also exist that support the commercial interests of companies, such as lobbying governments on behalf of pharmaceutical corporations, although it is not uncommon for them to hide their commercial agendas, thereby blurring boundaries between public and private (McCoy and Hilson 2009; Rowson 2005).

Civil society organizations are not, of course, a new type of actor; neither is their influence on health and other policies in democratic countries such as the UK a new thing. What is new is the dramatic increase in the number of CSOs operating at the global level and influencing global health policies and issues – up from 1983 in the early twentieth century to 37,000 in 2000 (McCoy and Hilson 2009, after Anheier et al. 2001). Hence we often hear the term *global* civil society being used to mean: 'the sphere of ideas, values, institutions, organisations, networks and individuals located *between* the family, the state, and the market and operating *beyond* the confines of national societies, polities, and economies' (Anheier et al. 2001, emphasis in original).

Globalization has both prompted and enabled the emergence of a global civil society. It has created and increased global health and social problems, many of which are beyond the control of country governments, such as global climate change, the transmission of global pandemics, and stark differences between rich and poor. Globalization also allows civil society organizations to operate at the global level because of easy access to the Internet and social media technologies enabling more extensive and immediate communication, such as the creation of 'transnational advocacy networks' working beyond national boundaries. There has also been a growth in global funding for health channelled through CSO implementers of health programmes in low- and middle-income countries (Rowson 2005).

 Activity 7.1

Make a list of health and other issues civil society organizations that have sought to influence health at the global level in recent decades.

Feedback

Civil society organizations have been involved in a vast number of issues including: gay rights; anti-poverty; anti-capitalism; cancelling unfair debt; global warming; universal access to health care; access to antiretroviral treatment; banning landmines; abortion laws; genetically modified crops; anti-deforestation; and mental health issues.

Global CSOs or international non-governmental organizations (INGOs) have influenced many important and contentious health issues. For example, they have played a key role in promoting breastfeeding by campaigning to establish an international code on the negative effects of infant formulas, known as the International Code for Marketing of Breast-milk Substitutes, and advocating for reduced tobacco consumption in low- and middle-income countries by contributing to the Framework Convention on Tobacco Control. Just as the term civil society captures many different types of organizations, the ways civil society organizations seek to influence global health are also diverse. Rowson (2005) provides a valuable typology of roles CSOs play in global health governance:

1 *Representing 'the voice of the people'*: advocating for the needs of marginalized and vulnerable groups, conveying or amplifying their expressed opinions and experiences, and supporting local people to directly participate in global debates.
2 *Advocacy and lobbying*: attempting to influence decisions through either confrontational means to challenge global institutions and their decisions, or consensual approaches involving participation and dialogue in shaping policy decisions.
3 *Research and policy analysis*: generating and sharing data on, for example, impacts of global decisions and policies.
4 *Watchdog*: independent monitoring and reporting on the policies and activities of global actors.
5 *Communication*: sharing information and communicating global policy decisions to promote transparency that can be especially important where information is shared between actors in low- and middle-income countries as well as those in high-income countries.
6 *Involvement in 'horizontal' governance mechanisms*: working with and forming alliances with global health actors through formal decision-making mechanisms.
7 *Involvement in multi-level governance*: participation together with national governments in global events and fora.
8 *Horizontal and vertical networking*: 'horizontal networking' with other non-governmental organizations and 'vertical networking' with government and multilateral agencies as ways to influence global health agendas.

9 *Building capacity of other civil society organizations*: typically northern CSOs supporting those in the South by providing resources, training, information, and contacts.

10 *Collaborating with global institutions in designing and implementing health interventions*: delivering health interventions as a way to reach poor, marginalized groups excluded from mainstream services and helping to inform government policy decisions about realities on the ground.

What is clear is that CSOs are increasingly shifting their stance from 'outsiders' targeting governments and other powerful health actors with advocacy campaigns, lobbying and acting as critical watchdogs, to 'insiders' partnering with other global health actors as members of governance mechanisms and networks (McCoy and Hilson 2009). Many CSOs are working with or are formally affiliated with UN agencies. For example, the WHO invites CSOs to input at technical working groups and committees that it convenes at global, regional, and country levels. Civil society organizations increasingly influence global health through participation in global health partnerships and in initiatives such as the Global Fund and the GAVI Alliance (Global Alliance for Vaccines and Immunization) alongside governments, UN agencies, and corporations. Indeed, their participation is increasingly formalized through having voting seats on decision-making boards, although some commentators suggest that this has increased corporations' influence on global health more than it has increased the influence of civil society on global health (Buse and Harmer 2007).

 Activity 7.2

Thinking about a country you are familiar with, make some notes on how increasing access to funding from bilateral donors and global health partnerships and initiatives might change civil society.

Feedback

There are several ways in which increasing access to funding may strengthen the ability of CSOs to influence health policies at national and global levels. Receiving donor funding may help them invest in management and financial systems, and this increasing professionalism can improve how governments and global actors perceive them. It can also enable them to travel to global meetings and conferences where they may have an influence on global-level decisions, and develop networks and alliances with other global actors.

Increasing dependence on funding from bilateral donors and global health partnerships and initiatives, however, leads some commentators to accuse funders of co-opting CSOs, leading the latter to compromise their values and weaken ties with the communities and groups they claim to represent. This may also mute their voices as they shift away from more critical advocacy or watchdog roles towards service provision.

Philanthropic foundations

Philanthropic foundations are a particular form of civil society organization (Owen et al. 2009), and can be defined as non-profit, non-governmental actors possessing a fund of their own, managed by trustees and directors and promoting public welfare, including social, educational, charitable, religious or other activities (Scott et al. 2003). However, it can be difficult to differentiate between foundations and other non-profit, non-governmental organizations, in part because the term is often used interchangeably with 'endowment', 'trust' or 'fund' and captures diverse types of actors that include private and public foundations, corporate foundations, single social entrepreneurs, venture philanthropists, and 'philanthrocapitalists'.

When talking about philanthropic foundations and global health, we usually think of the Bill and Melinda Gates Foundation, established in the 1990s, not least because of its substantial annual grants totalling over US$3 billion. With a large contribution in 2006 from Warren Buffet, a US investor and philanthropist, worth over US$30 billion, it became the largest private donor to the WHO and the second largest donor overall after the US Government. There are other well-known foundations, and many of the largest are from the USA, such as the Rockefeller Foundation (established 1913) and the Ford Foundation (established 1936), and from the UK, including the Carnegie Foundation (established 1905) and the Wellcome Trust (established 1936). Such foundations are clearly not new; neither is their ability to influence global health. The Rockefeller Foundation, for instance, played an important role in establishing the League of Nations Health Organization, including providing 40 per cent of the organization's original budget (see also the discussion in Chapter 4) (Birn and Fee 2013).

Among the advantages that foundations have over traditional bilateral and multilateral global health actors is their relative freedom to promote innovative approaches to health and other development issues. They are often able to draw attention to issues that are not emphasized by traditional actors, and are freer than other actors to criticize governments and pressurize them to act. Large foundations are becoming important global health actors, much of their influence stemming from their substantial contributions to development assistance for health over the last decade.

The Gates Foundation with its large contributions to the WHO and the Global Fund is widely credited with injecting energy into global health and increasing global attention on diseases such as malaria and polio (*The Lancet* 2009). It is a key member of a number of global partnerships and networks, including Roll Back Malaria and the Global Alliance for Improved Nutrition, and Gates funding of US$750 million helped establish the GAVI Alliance in 2000 (Buse and Harmer 2009). The foundation is even a member of 'H8', an elite group of global health actors that includes the World Bank and the health-related UN agencies, the GAVI Alliance and the Global Fund, and was a signatory of the International Health Partnership global compact in 2007 (Owen et al. 2009).

Global health partnerships and initiatives

Global health partnerships (GHPs), a term often used interchangeably with global public private partnerships (GPPPs) and sometimes global health initiatives (GHIs), captures a range of financing, coordinating, and implementing entities that are diverse in their functions, size, and scope. Some focus on a specific health problem or disease, others on research and development of or donation of new drugs, vaccines or other products, or working on broader health systems issues, raising consciousness through campaigning and advocacy, technical assistance, or health service and system support (Buse and Harmer 2009; Buse and Walt 2000).

The urgent need to address persistent and newly emerging global health threats such as HIV and AIDS meant that new thinking was required to harness the energy, business skills, innovative ideas and expertise, and financial resources of partnerships of traditional and new actors – including civil society and foundations as well as businesses such as pharmaceutical corporations (Buse et al. 2005; Walt et al. 2009). Hence, many global health partnerships and initiatives were created in the late 1980s, 1990s, and early 2000s and have become 'part of mainstream global health discourse and a dominant model for cooperation in a complex world' (Buse and Harmer 2009: 245). The WHO Maximizing Positive Synergies Collaborative Group (2009) lists 100 GHPs and GHIs with involvement of several stakeholders covering health issues as diverse as HIV/AIDS, malaria, tuberculosis, vaccines, drugs for neglected tropical diseases, schistosomiasis, diarrhoea control, handwashing, and reproductive health to name a few.

Some of the largest and best-known GHPs and GHIs include the Global Fund to Fight AIDS, Tuberculosis and Malaria, the GAVI Alliance, and the President's Emergency Plan for AIDS Relief (PEPFAR). These and others have mobilized substantial additional funding for health programmes. Such funding equates to a considerable proportion of overall development aid for health in many low- and middle-income countries, and in some cases external funding from GHPs and GHIs for HIV/AIDS exceeds domestic budgets for health as a whole. This has led to a dramatic scaling up of HIV/AIDS programmes and has improved access to services for populations with a limited ability to pay (Buse and Harmer 2007; Walt et al. 2009).

The GHPs and GHIs are credited with raising the profile of particular health issues on national and international policy agendas, strengthening country policy processes and health delivery capacity, and establishing international norms and standards (Buse and Harmer 2007). They have also brought some consensus among different partners with diverse interests, although this consensus has been delicate (Walt et al. 2009). There has been broad agreement about the urgent need to mobilize substantial resources for programmes to tackle HIV/AIDS, particularly in the countries of east and southern Africa. However, differences between two of the biggest GHIs – the Global Fund and PEPFAR – illustrate a lack of agreement about the best approach to doing this. The Global Fund, with its complex multi-partner governance arrangements, finances recipient country proposals for the three focal diseases and channels funds through a mix of government and CSO implementers via a 'Principal Recipient'. PEPFAR, on the other hand, is a bilateral HIV/AIDS programme of the US Government that adopts a more prescriptive approach, and aims at rapid results by channelling the bulk of its funding through CSO recipients.

Activity 7.3

Can you think of other major global health partnerships and initiatives? Make a short list of those that come to mind. Now list their main focus of activities. That is, do they address a specific set of diseases such as HIV or malaria, or an issue such as immunization or child health?

Feedback

Some of the best-known global health partnerships and initiatives include:

- World Bank's Multi-country AIDS Program (MAP)
- Stop Tuberculosis Partnership
- Roll Back Malaria (RBM)
- Global Alliance for Improved Nutrition (GAIN)
- International AIDS Vaccine Initiative (IAVI)

You may have listed other global health partnerships and initiatives, and there may be some initiatives that address the same or overlapping issues. This gives a sense of how 'crowded' the space in global health is today.

Challenges: more actors = better health governance?

Harmonization and alignment

The explosion in the numbers of new global actors – 'a dazzling kaleidoscopic environment' according to Walt et al. (2009) – creates important challenges for global health actors and the countries receiving aid for health. The problem is fragmentation: poor co-ordination among global health actors and implementers ('harmonization') and between external programmes and recipient government policies, programmes, systems, and targets ('alignment'). Such problems are fuelled by competing priorities and mandates among donors and other global health actors, donor governments' national security, economic and foreign policy interests, competition for donor funding among implementers, and pressure to attribute outcomes to programmatic efforts while delivering results to ambitious time-frames (Shorten et al. 2012).

Poor harmonization and alignment have damaging effects on recipient countries with fragile health systems. Donors, including GHPs and GHIs, often introduce parallel monitoring/evaluation and financial management procedures and duplicate coordination mechanisms, adding to already complex governance arrangements that place a considerable burden on recipient country governments. Like many bilateral health programmes before them, many of the GHPs and GHIs have introduced 'vertical' programmes (focusing on specific health issues) rather than broad, 'horizontal' primary healthcare interventions, which are criticized for imposing external priorities on recipient countries leading to a skewing of national policies and reducing 'country ownership' – the power and influence of recipient governments to determine their own policies and priorities (Biesma et al. 2009; Buse and Harmer 2007; Spicer and Harmer 2014; Spicer et al, 2010; WHO Maximizing Positive Synergies Collaborative Group 2009). Sridhar (2010: 460) sums up these issues:

> the current [global health] landscape is characterized by fragmentation, lack of coordination, and even confusion as a diverse array of well-funded and well-meaning initiatives descend with good intentions on countries in the developing world.

Several high-profile declarations and initiatives signal global recognition of the problems of aid effectiveness, including the Paris Declaration of Aid Effectiveness (2005), which proposes principles of more predictable, longer-term aid commitments, improved harmonization and alignment, and better government ownership of externally funded programmes among others. Shorten et al. (2012) list no less than nineteen major aid effectiveness declarations, initiatives, and processes since the 1980s demonstrating sustained global resolve, but also revealing that despite these efforts the problems of aid effectiveness do not appear to be diminishing, thereby raising questions about whether global commitments are reflected in practices on the ground.

Accountability and legitimacy

While many commentators welcome the shifts in power and influence the growth of global civil society represents, this uncoordinated 'swarm' of global CSOs is viewed by some as a potential threat to the dominance of governments, UN agencies, and transnational corporations. One criticism relates to whether CSOs are accountable in the same way as country governments are to voters, citizens, and taxpayers, and the extent to which they are democratic. Democracy enables civil society to exist, and the existence of civil society can strengthen democracy through its ability to challenge and hold powerful governments, and indeed transnational corporations and multilateral agencies, to account. However, unlike (many) national governments, CSOs are not democratically elected: they do not represent populations in the same ways as governments, and some commentators point to parallels between large North CSO and colonial administrators and missionaries imposing ideas and values on southern governments (Doyle and Patel 2008). Indeed, while funding from donors and foundations may empower and enable CSOs to act at the global level, this may weaken links to the poor, marginalized groups they claim to represent – and lines of accountability may be stronger to funders than communities (McCoy and Hilson 2009; Spicer et al. 2011). With increasing global funding being channelled through CSO health programme implementers, and thereby bypassing governments, the ability of the latter to build and maintain its own democratic legitimacy may be undermined (Doyle and Patel 2008).

The problems of a lack of accountability and legitimacy may be particularly problematic in the case of some of the largest foundations, such as the Bill and Melinda Gates Foundation, which have substantial power to influence decisions at global and country level derived from their huge resources. At the same time, they lack the formal public accountability mechanisms of most governments and UN agencies. According to Reich (2002: 4), such foundations have 'too much power to set public agendas, without sufficient public oversight and input'. While the Gates Foundation is widely credited with energizing and raising the profile of global health issues, critics have pointed to the Foundation's lack of transparency and limited involvement of other actors in its decision-making, poor alignment of its grant-making with country health priorities, and the fact that it channels the bulk of its funding through US and other northern CSO implementers thereby sidelining smaller southern CSOs and recipient governments.

Foundations have also been criticized for potential conflicts of interest. Among some of the larger foundations there are significant investments in pharmaceutical and food corporations, overlapping board directorships with these corporations, and examples of partnership arrangements where corporations potentially benefit from foundations' tax-exempt status. The Gates Foundation is a major shareholder of the Coca-Cola Corporation, which it has supported to develop new supply chains. Critics argue that while there are clear links between consumption of sugary drinks and rises in diabetes and obesity (which are overtaking infectious diseases in low- and middle-income countries), the Foundation's investments in these health issues have been very low (Stuckler et al. 2011). There have been calls for foundations to improve accountability and transparency, to focus investments on strengthening health systems rather than commodities and technologies, and to place more emphasis than they currently do on the most important global health issues (*The Lancet* 2007, 2009; McCoy et al. 2009; Sridhar and Batniji 2008; Stuckler et al. 2011).

Power and money

As well as being heterogeneous in their type and roles, CSOs are very diverse in size. Well-known northern CSOs such as Médecins sans Frontières, Oxfam, and Save the Children are highly professionalized and well-resourced in contrast to the multitude of smaller CSOs, especially those based in the Global South. As well as far greater capacity and resources, the former have far better access to and influence at the global level than the latter. Indeed, many smaller, southern-based CSOs lack the capacity and resources to engage in global-level discussions, which often involve attending meetings in Geneva or Washington. The ability of large, well-funded northern CSOs to represent the views and needs of poor, marginalized groups in the South has been questioned by some commentators who suggest they are more in tune with dominant ideas about globalization and global health than potentially more critical ideas and perspectives of marginalized groups (Doyle and Patel 2008; McCoy and Hilson 2009).

Another concern relates to the potential for co-option of CSOs by bilateral donors and foundations resulting in shifts away from advocacy or watchdog roles to implementing health programmes. While this has professionalized some CSOs and enabled them to work alongside government and development partners, it may also mute their ability to challenge and hold governments and other powerful actors to account on controversial issues such as drug use, sex work, and HIV/AIDS (Doyle and Patel 2008; Harmer et al. 2013; Spicer et al. 2011). In Chapter 6, we also explore how commercial sector actors use and co-opt CSOs.

Summary

In this chapter, you have learnt about the diversity of civil society organizations, philanthropic foundations, and global health partnerships and initiatives, and assessed the increasing significance of these 'new' actors in decision-making at the global level. You also explored some key challenges: problems of coordinating the increasing numbers of global health actors; problems of civil society organizations and foundations maintaining accountability and legitimacy; and the imbalances between large northern and small southern civil society organizations in terms of their influence on global health decisions.

References

Anheier, H., Glasius, M. and Kaldor, M. (2001) Introducing global society, in H. Anheier, M. Glasius and M. Kaldor (eds) *Global Civil Society 2001*. New York: Oxford University Press.

Biesma, R., Brugha, R., Harmer, A., Walsh, A., Spicer, N. and Walt, G. (2009) The effects of global HIV/AIDS initiatives on country health systems: a review of the evidence, *Health Policy and Planning*, 24 (4): 239–52.

Birn, A.-E. and Fee, E. (2013) The Rockefeller Foundation and the international health agenda, *The Lancet*, 381 (9878): 1618–19.

Buse, K. and Harmer, A. (2007) Seven habits of highly effective global public–private health partnerships: practice and potential, *Social Science and Medicine*, 64 (2): 259–71.

Buse, K. and Harmer, A. (2009) Global health partnerships: the mosh pit of global health governance, in K. Buse, W. Hein and N. Drager (eds) *Making Sense of Global Health Governance: A Policy Perspective*. Basingstoke: Palgrave Macmillan.

Buse, K., Mays, N. and Walt, G. (2005) *Making Health Policy*. Maidenhead: McGraw-Hill.

Buse, K. and Walt, G. (2000) Global public–private partnerships: part I – a new development in health?, *Bulletin of the World Health Organization*, 78 (4): 549–61.

Dodd, R., Schieber, G., Cassels, A., Fleisher, L. and Gorret, P. (2007) Aid effectiveness and health. Making Health Systems Work: Working Paper No. 9. Geneva: World Health Organization.

Doyle, C. and Patel, P. (2008) Civil society organizations and global health initiatives: problems of legitimacy, *Social Science and Medicine*, 66: 1928–38.

Harmer, A., Spicer, N., Bogdan, D., Chkhatarashvili, K., Murzalieva, G., Rukhadze, N. et al. (2013) Has Global Fund support of civil society advocacy in the former Soviet Union established meaningful engagement or 'a lot of jabber about nothing'?, *Health Policy and Planning*, 28 (3): 299–308.

IHME (2009) *Financing Global Health 2009: Tracking Development Assistance for Health*. Seattle, WA: Institute for Health Metrics and Evaluation.

Lancet (2007) Editorial: Governance questions at the Gates Foundation, *The Lancet*, 369: 163.

Lancet (2009) Editorial: What has the Gates Foundation done for global health?, *The Lancet*, 373: 1577.

McCoy, D. and Hilson, M. (2009) Civil society, its organizations, and global health governance, in K. Buse, W. Hein and N. Drager (eds) *Making Sense of Global Health Governance: A Policy Perspective*. Basingstoke: Palgrave Macmillan.

McCoy, D., Kembhavi, G., Patel, J. and Luintel, A. (2009) The Bill & Melinda Gates Foundation's grant-making programme for global health, *The Lancet*, 373: 1645–53.

Owen, J., Lister, G. and Stansfield, S. (2009) The role of foundations in global governance for health, in K. Buse, W. Hein and N. Drager (eds) *Making Sense of Global Health Governance: A Policy Perspective*. Basingstoke: Palgrave Macmillan.

Reich, M.R. (2002) Introduction: public–private partnerships for public health, in M.R. Reich (ed.) *Public–Private Partnerships for Public Health*, pp. 1–18. Cambridge, MA: Harvard Center for Population and Development Studies.

Rowson, M. (2005) Health and an emerging civil society, in K. Lee and J. Collin (eds) *Global Change and Health*. Maidenhead: Open University Press.

Scott, S., Adelman, C., Sebag, R. and Asenjo Ruiz, C. (2003) Philanthropic foundations and development cooperation, *DAC Journal*, 4 (3): 73–148.

Shorten, T., Taylor, M., Spicer, N., Mounier-Jack, S. and McCoy, D. (2012) The *International Health Partnership Plus*: rhetoric or real change? Results of a self-reported survey in the run-up to the 4th High Level Forum on Aid Effectiveness in Busan, *Globalization and Health*, 8: 13.

Spicer, N., Aleshkina, J., Biesma, R., Brugha, R., Caceres, C., Chilundo, B. et al. (2010) National and sub-national HIV/AIDS coordination: are global health initiatives closing the gap between intent and practice?, *Globalization and Health*, 6: 3.

Spicer, N. and Harmer, A. (2014) Global health initiatives and financing for health, in A.J. Culyer (ed.) *Encyclopedia of Health Economics*. London: Elsevier.

Spicer, N., Harmer, A., Bogdan, D., Chkhatarashvili, K., Murzalieva, G., Rukhadze, N. et al. (2011) Circus monkeys or change agents? Civil society advocacy for HIV/AIDS in adverse policy environments, *Social Science and Medicine*, 73 (12): 1748–55.

Sridhar, D. (2010) Seven challenges in international development assistance for health and ways forward, *Journal of Law, Medicine and Ethics*, 38 (3): 459–69.

Sridhar, D. and Batniji, R. (2008) Misfinancing global health: a case for transparency in disbursements and decision making, *The Lancet*, 372: 1185–91.

Stuckler, D., Basu, S. and McKee, M. (2011) Global health philanthropy and institutional relationships: how should conflicts of interest be addressed?, *PLoS Medicine*, 8(4): e1001020.

UN (2004) *We the Peoples: Civil Society, the United Nations and Global Governance*. Report of the Panel of Eminent Persons on United Nations–Civil Society Relations. New York: United Nations.

Walt, G., Spicer, N. and Buse, K. (2009) Mapping the global health architecture, in K. Buse, W. Hein and N. Drager (eds) *Making Sense of Global Health Governance: A Policy Perspective*. Basingstoke: Palgrave Macmillan.

World Health Organization Maximizing Positive Synergies Collaborative Group (2009) An assessment of interactions between global health initiatives and country health systems, *The Lancet*, 373 (9681): 2137–69.

8 Trade and global health

Helen Walls, Johanna Hanefeld, Richard Smith, Nick Drager and Kelley Lee

Overview

In this chapter, we will learn about trade policy and, in particular, the potential implications of multilateral, regional, and bilateral trade agreements for public health. We will cover the history of the international trading system, basic principles underpinning trade law, and the key trade agreements governing trade today, including the role of the World Trade Organization (WTO). We will consider the relevance, in particular, of the Agreement on Trade Related Intellectual Property Rights (TRIPS) and the General Agreement on Trade in Services (GATS) for public health. We will also address the need for regulatory capacity and coordination to manage opportunities and risks associated with trade agreements.

Learning objectives

After working through this chapter, you will be able to:

- describe the origins, structure, and functions of the WTO, and the multilateral trade agreements under its remit
- understand the broad ways in which trade issues can be relevant to public health
- understand the basic parameters of the TRIPS and GATS Agreements and their potential relevance to public health
- appreciate the need for regulatory capacity and coordination to manage risks associated with trade agreements

Key terms

Compulsory licence: The permission given by a government to a third party to use or produce an invention without the consent of the patent holder. *For patents*: when the authorities license companies or individuals other than the patent owner to use the rights of the patent – to make, use, sell or import a product under patent (i.e. a patented product or a product made by a patented process) – without the permission of the patent owner. Allowed under the WTO's TRIPS (intellectual property) Agreement provided certain procedures and conditions are fulfilled.

Most favoured nation principle: In a trade agreement between two countries, if either party to the treaty grants a favour (usually a tariff reduction) to a third country, the other party to the treaty will be granted the same favour: what is given to one is given to all.

Non-tariff barrier: Barriers to trade that are either quota or quantitative restrictions deliberately designed to protect domestic industries, or internal taxes, administrative requirements, health and sanitary regulations, and government procurement policies that are not necessarily intended to restrict trade.

Parallel import: The importation of a product without the approval of the owner of patent or trademark or copyright. When a product made legally (i.e. not pirated) abroad is imported without the permission of the intellectual property right-holder (e.g. the trademark or patent owner).

Tariff: A tax levied against an imported good (or service).

Introduction

International trade should lead to improved economic growth, lower cost, and wider access to goods and services through the reduction of trade barriers. Trade liberalization – often as a result of negotiations of bilateral, regional, and global trade agreements – can affect health in multiple ways (WHO/WTO 2002). Sometimes the effect is obvious, as when a disease crosses borders together with a traded good. On other occasions, the effects of trade liberalization are more indirect. For example, reducing tariffs may lead to lower prices for medical equipment and health-related products; changing international rules concerning patent protection may affect the prices of medicines and vaccines (Smith et al. 2009a).

Global trade increases the availability of products such as alcohol, tobacco, and processed foods that influence the prevalence of non-communicable disease. The promotion and advertising of harmful substances, such as tobacco and alcohol, are also often regulated through trade agreements. Trade in health services, including the provision of health services across borders, and the movement of human resources for health from one country to another, also affects health systems, and may impact on the cost, access to, and quality of health services available for the local population. As trade liberalization creates both opportunities and risks for health, there is a need for greater interaction between trade and health policy-makers and practitioners and greater mutual awareness of trade and health policies.

The signing of trade agreements also has important implications for public health. Trade agreements may have implications for equity within and between countries, and for public health, through their impact on factors such as access to pharmaceuticals, and the ability of states to regulate on public health grounds. In fact, it is argued that clauses recently included in trade agreements may restrict domestic policy-making space and have implications for national sovereignty. To understand this better, it is important to understand the history of international trade.

A brief history of the world trading system

Trade has occurred between societies throughout human history, with rules governing trade relations becoming more formalized as societies have developed. Trade was initially by barter, the direct exchange of goods and services. Later, traders generally negotiated through a medium of exchange – money. A more recent development has been the introduction of tariff barriers to trade, whereby trading parties may impose taxes on imports to encourage or discourage the trade of certain goods; usually to protect or favour a domestic producer. During the eighteenth century, principles were developed among leading trading nations to facilitate the cross-border movement of goods. Perhaps the most important is the most favoured nation (MFN) principle, which states that in a trade agreements between two countries, if either party to the treaty grants a favour (usually a tariff reduction) to a third country, then the other party to the treaty will be granted that same favour. The First World War (1914–19), and events thereafter, led to a weakening of the application of this principle. This is often suggested to have resulted in the escalating and punitive application of tariffs by many governments and caused a major depression in the world economy, eventually culminating in the Second World War.

After the Second World War, efforts were therefore made to create a new system of international trade that would prevent 'tit-for-tat' protectionism from again threatening peace and stability. The original plan was to create a permanent International Trade Organization (ITO), as agreed in Havana, Cuba, in 1948. As an institution, the proposed ITO would rank alongside the World Bank and International Monetary Fund. Its work would be based around a General Agreement on Trade and Tariffs (GATT), signed by 23 states in 1947, as part of efforts to create a more stable world economy. However, the ITO was not established. The US Government declined to ratify its charter and the GATT became, by default, the only multilateral agreement governing world trade.

The GATT institutional framework became the driving force behind trade liberalization over the next fifty years. It served as the forum for negotiating reductions in tariffs through a series of 'trade rounds' held between 1947 and 1994. Table 8.1 lists these trade rounds, the number of countries participating, and trade concessions achieved. Note the growth in number of countries involved, the broadened scope of subjects under negotiation, and, not unrelated, the length of time taken for rounds to conclude.

GATT was successful. Since 1945, average tariffs have plummeted and international trade has rapidly increased in scale and scope. A wave of trade liberalization occurred from the 1970s to mid-1990s, with a particular increase in the signing of bilateral

Table 8.1 Trade rounds held under the GATT, 1947–94

Trade round	No. of participant countries	Subject of negotiations
Geneva Round (1947)	23	Concessions on 43 tariff lines
Annecy Round (1949)	29	Modest reductions
Torquay Round (1950–51)	32	8700 concessions
Geneva Round (1955–56)	33	Modest reductions
Dillon Round (1960–61)	39	Formation of EEC 4400 concessions
Kennedy Round (1963–67)	74	Anti-dumping, customs valuation, preferential treatment to less-developed countries
Tokyo Round (1973–79)	99	1/3 tariff reduction by developed countries, codes of conduct on non-tariff barriers
Uruguay Round (1986–94)	124	1/3 tariff reduction by by developed countries, agriculture, clothing, GATS, TRIPS, WTO created
Doha Round (2001–)	155	Tariff reductions, agriculture and a number of other areas

Source: Trading Economics (2013).

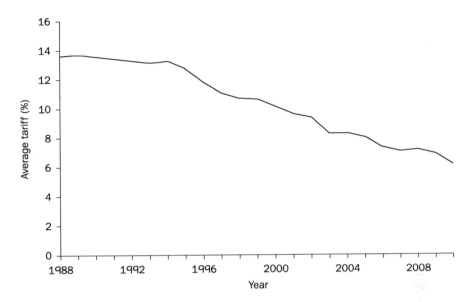

Figure 8.1 Average tariff rate, all products (%) globally

(between two countries) and regional (within geographical region) trade agreements (RTAs), including the North American Free Trade Agreement (NAFTA), the Asian Free Trade Agreement (AFTA), the European Union (EU) and the Andean Common Market (ANCOM). The US was the most sought-after bilateral trade partner, given the size of its import market. These TAs contributed to a reduction in tariffs (Figure 8.1), which fell on average from around 40% in 1940 to 4% in 1995. Consequently, cross-border trade (measured by the ratio of world trade to world output or national trade to GDP minus government expenditure) has intensified. There has also been an increase in the number of countries involved in the international trading system.

The creation of the World Trade Organization

The most significant trade round of GATT was the Uruguay Round, which lasted almost eight years (1986–94). Its conclusion led to the replacement of the GATT with the World Trade Organization (WTO) in 1995. Since this time especially, trade liberalization, which used to be about removing tariff barriers to trade in goods, has begun to cover areas not formerly part of the trade regime. Trade rules under the WTO expanded to cover services and intellectual property rights, for example.

The WTO's stated functions are to do the following:

- serve as a forum for trade negotiations, monitoring national trade policies, and settling trade disputes;
- carry out day-to-day administration of trade agreements under its jurisdiction;
- assist member states in implementing trade agreements; and
- oversee special arrangements for low-income countries in their compliance with trade agreements.

The latter, however, does not mean that WTO is a funding body. Indeed, it has no mandate to finance development projects. Rather, the organization provides special and preferential treatment to low-income countries in the form of exemptions from certain obligations or reciprocity, longer transition periods, and technical assistance. For example, it offers training to officials in understanding the trading system, administration of agreements, and taking effective part in trade negotiations.

The WTO currently (2013) has 157 member states. Together, they account for more than 90 per cent of world trade. But this figure excludes a huge 'informal' or parallel economy including the global trade in illicit drugs, counterfeit goods, and people trafficking, all of which have health-related consequences. Membership of the WTO is not automatic, requiring negotiation with existing member states. After a membership application is submitted, a working party is set up by the General Council (see Figure 8.2), which, while open to all member states, usually consists of those countries with an interest in the applicant country's trade regime. The applicant government presents a memorandum covering all aspects of its trade and legal regime to the working party. At the same time, the applicant government engages in bilateral negotiations with interested working party members on concessions and commitments on market access for goods and services. The results of these bilateral negotiations are consolidated into a document that is part of the final 'accession package'. The entire process can take several years, with China's accession in 2001 taking 14 years of negotiation. With so many countries now members, there is pressure to join for any country seeking to trade.

The WTO is based in Geneva with about 500 staff, headed by a Director-General (Figure 8.2). Its top decision-making body is the Ministerial Conference, which brings together leading trade officials of member states at least once every two years. The General Council meets several times a year in Geneva and is attended by ambassadors, representatives of countries with permanent trade delegations in Geneva, and officials from member states (which may include health experts). The General Council also meets as the Trade Policy Review Body and the Dispute Settlement Body. The annual budget of the WTO is around US$220 million.

The overall principles underpinning the world trading system under the WTO are:

- most favoured nation treatment;
- trade without discrimination;
- use of tariffs to ensure predictable and increased access to markets;
- promotion of fair competition;
- encouragement of development and economic reform; and
- transparency.

These principles are set out in the GATT (for goods), and the General Agreement on Trade in Services (for services). Additional agreements deal with the special requirements of specific sectors or issues. Some have detailed and lengthy schedules (or lists) of commitments made by individual countries. In services, for example, the commitments state how much access a foreign-service provider is allowed for a specific sector.

One important innovation of the WTO is the creation of a new procedure for settling trade disputes. Formal dispute settlement is an option of last resort. Nevertheless, if two or more WTO members have a dispute over a trade measure and cannot resolve it between themselves (or in other fora), they have the right to bring the dispute to the Dispute Settlement Body (DSB) of the WTO (the General Council in another guise). A dispute can only be brought between member states, and only about alleged failures to comply with WTO agreements or commitments. Companies, organizations, and private individuals cannot complain directly to the WTO, but can do so through a member state. When a dispute

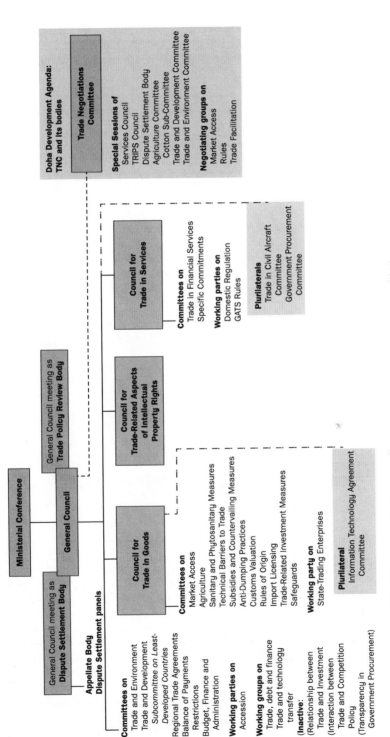

Figure 8.2 Structure of the World Trade Organization

Source: WTO (2013)

is lodged, a panel of experts is established by the DSB to consider the case. The WTO then has the sole authority to accept or reject the panel's findings or the results of an appeal. It monitors implementation of rulings and recommendations from panels and the Appellate Body. It also has the power to authorize compensation or suspension of concessions if a country fails to comply with a ruling.

Further developments in trade

The most significant influence on international trade policy has come from the rules set out by the World Trade Organisation (WTO), that focus on enabling easier trade for its 157 current member countries. However, the latest round of WTO negotiations – the Doha Round, launched in 2001 and targeting further trade liberalization and integration of developing countries into global trade – has stalled. A particular issue of contention is the maintenance of developed countries' agricultural subsidies, seen to operate effectively as trade barriers. Farmers in the USA and the EU, for example, receive substantial subsidies for their production, without which they would be far less competitive against producers from low-income countries. As a result of this breakdown of the WTO negotiations, increasingly significant influence in world trade is also coming from regional and bilateral trade agreements (RTAs). There are currently (as of 2013) 261 notified to the WTO.

 Activity 8.1

In your home, can you find ten items that have been imported from other countries? How many items can you find imported from different continents? Is there one country or region where most of your imported goods come from?

Feedback

It should not be difficult to find imported goods in your home. Most are likely to come from countries or regions that have special trading relationships with your home country, or from countries that led the world in manufacturing such as China and the USA.

Protection of trade versus public health

While historical precedent and powerful vested interests have given substantial weight to international trade law, there have been efforts to balance its application with other policy objectives including public health. For example, a notable exception to the most favoured nation principle is that a member state may restrict trade on goods and/or services when necessary to protect the health of humans, animals, and plants on the condition that either the restriction is applied in a non-discriminatory way or the restriction is based on recognized scientific evidence (Article XX, GATT). Article XVI of the General Agreement on Trade in Services (see below) authorizes a similar restriction on services and service suppliers (Blouin et al. 2006; Smith et al. 2009b).

The first requirement suggests that, if the intention is to protect the consumer, it should not matter where the health risk originates. This does not mean that if a government allows imports of a particular product from one country, it must allow imports of the same product from all countries. For example, the same fish product might be allowed in from one country but banned from another because it is contaminated with cholera. The same requirement must apply to all countries, but will affect them differently depending on the health status of their product.

The second requirement means that a trade restriction cannot be a disguised form of protectionism. Measures taken to restrict trade must be no more than is necessary. There is no requirement under Article XX of GATT to quantify the risk to human life or health. To determine whether a restrictive measure is necessary requires a weighing and balancing of factors that include:

• the importance of the interests protected by the measure;
• the efficacy of such measure in pursuing the policies; and
• the impact of the law or regulation on imports or exports.

There are examples of disputes arising from trade restrictions in an effort to protect public health. A WTO member state can challenge the imposition of such measures through the Dispute Settlement Body (described above) if it feels there are unfair trade practices at play. Evidence sustaining the restrictive measure must be of recognized scientific standards, and the use of the so-called 'precautionary principle' to avert potential versus proven risk/harm to health (as you will see in Chapter 10), as a basis for limiting trade, remains subject to dispute. A good example is food imports. A country may decide, for instance, to restrict an imported fruit because of what it deems an unacceptable level of pesticide presence. This is a legitimate public health concern and, if applied in a non-discriminatory way (i.e. to all member states) and based on scientific principles (research shows this to be a risk), it is a justifiable trade barrier under WTO rules. A dispute can arise where the scientific evidence is unclear or contentious. The dispute between the European Community and US Government over the import of hormone-treated beef into EC member states arose from disagreement over the scientific evidence on the true risk. The dispute arose in 1988 when the EC prohibited the use of hormonal substances for animal growth promotion, including 17β oestradiol, testosterone, progesterone, zeranol, trenbolone acetate, and melengestrol acetate. The ban applies without discrimination internally and to all imports from third countries from 1 January 1989. Third countries wishing to export bovine meat and meat products to the EU had to either have equivalent legislation or to operate a hormone-free cattle programme. Some 90 per cent of US cattle producers routinely use hormones to make cattle grow faster and bigger. After the ban was imposed, the US exported only hormone-free beef to the EU, losing an estimated US$500 million annually. A series of trade sanctions have been imposed by the US and Canada in response. The EU prohibition has been maintained despite two rulings that it does not comply with WTO commitments, and the EU has sought to reopen the issue at the DSB/WTO based on new evidence. The WTO ruling that the EU had to remove the import ban led to criticisms of the expertise used to assess the risk, and the scope permitting application of the precautionary principle. In contrast, a dispute between the EU and Canadian Government over the banning in 1997 of imported asbestos by the French Government resulted in an upholding of the import ban by the WTO in 2000 on the grounds of protecting public health (WTO 2001). These two cases demonstrate that, while the WTO provides scope to protect public health, this is strongly dependent on the availability of 'clear' scientific evidence.

A future area of dispute is likely to be trade in goods and services that are inherently harmful to health. Tobacco products are perhaps the best example but one might also include the international arms trade and toxic waste. According to the economic theory of David Ricardo, free trade generally leads to increased competition, improved efficiency, and lower prices. All of these factors, in turn, lead to increased production and consumption of the traded product. This is assumed to be beneficial when concerned with 'goods'. However, public health advocates argue that tobacco and other products should be considered 'bads', with increased production and consumption leading to greater harm in the form of greater death and disease. Evidence shows that trade liberalization of tobacco products has led to an increase in consumption, and thus an adverse health impact, in low-income countries. The tobacco industry has actively lobbied in bilateral, regional, and multilateral trade forums for its products to be treated like any other good. Public health advocates argue that tobacco should be treated differently, allowing countries to restrict its trade. This is likely to be an important area of tension between trade and health in forthcoming trade negotiations. Equally and as discussed in Chapter 6 on private sector actors, tobacco companies have attempted to use provisions set out in international trade agreements to avoid stricter regulation, including plain packaging.

Importantly for public health, new RTAs under negotiation such as the Trans Pacific Partnership (TPP) involving a number of Asia-Pacific countries, including the USA, are likely to include unprecedented clauses, providing strong investor protections, which would introduce vast changes to regulatory regimes to enable greater industry involvement in policy-making and new avenues for appeal. These new clauses may undermine domestic policy-making space, making it difficult for states to legislate in favour of public health. This includes regulations and standards, such as health and safety.

An additional example is the US request for 'TRIPS plus' provisions on intellectual property in RTAs such as the TPP. The Agreement on Trade Related Aspects of Intellectual Property (TRIPS) will be discussed in more detail in the next section. In 2001, at the ministerial meeting of the WTO in Doha, Qatar, the 'Doha Declaration' reaffirmed countries' right to use TRIPS safeguards such as compulsory licences or parallel importation to overcome patent barriers to promote access to medicines, and guided countries in their use. Despite the Doha Declaration, in recent years developing countries have come under pressure to enact even tougher or more restrictive conditions in their patent laws than are required by the TRIPS agreement – these are known as the 'TRIPS Plus' provisions. While the US has been heavily criticized for requesting TRIPS Plus provisions on intellectual property in the TPP, this has not resulted in any change.

One of the challenges in negotiations of trade agreements is the varying levels of capacity and resources available to high-, middle-, and low-income countries. Studies of trade agreements between large developed countries and small developing countries have found that the small country often gives up a lot in order to gain a little. When multinational corporations (MNCs) become (directly or indirectly) involved in trade negotiations, not only are trade negotiations between countries unequal regards levels of bargaining power, they are also much more unequal depending on where MNCs throw their weight.

🖉 **Activity 8.2**

Make a list of goods and services that you think might pose a direct risk to public health if traded from one country to another. Describe how such a risk might emerge.

Feedback

Some examples of goods include tobacco products, contaminated foodstuffs, toxic chemicals, and military weapons. Examples of potentially risky services are unregulated health services, such as alternative therapies, or inappropriate advertising messages. Think about potential health risks that may arise from the time a good or service arrives into the country, to their purchase and use by the end consumer.

Agreement on Trade Related Intellectual Property Rights (TRIPS) and access to medicines

A relatively new feature of the WTO, not present under GATT, was the Agreement on Trade Related Aspects of Intellectual Property Rights (TRIPS) adopted at the end of the Uruguay Round in 1995. The agreement sets out minimum standards for protecting and enforcing nearly all forms of intellectual property rights (i.e. patents, trademarks, and copyright) for member states. All member states must comply with these standards, where necessary modifying their national legislation. Importantly, the agreement (Article 8) explicitly acknowledges that, in framing national laws, members 'may . . . adopt measures necessary to protect public health and nutrition, and to promote the public interest'.

In an important departure from previous conventions, pharmaceutical products are accorded full intellectual property rights (IPR) under TRIPS. Pharmaceutical companies are granted the legal means, as patent owners of new drug products, to prevent others from making, using or selling the new invention for a limited period of time. The TRIPS agreement specifies that patents must be available for all discoveries that 'are new, involve an inventive step and are capable of industrial application' (Article 27). Patent protection can thus be obtained for new drug products that enable the patent holder to have exclusive rights to produce and sell the product. Pharmaceutical companies argue that such rights, and the consequent ability to charge a higher price for a drug under patent, are necessary to recoup the many millions of dollars spent to research and develop the drug, and bring it to market.

Without the prospect of earning such prices, the incentive to invest in research and development (R&D) would be seriously undermined (WTO 2003). However, other authors (notably Light and Warburton 2011) refute such claims, suggesting that high R&D cost estimates have been constructed by industry-supported economists, and providing evidence that pharmaceutical companies fund a fairly small fraction of R&D (with the majority of drug discovery research instead funded by government and public sources), while most of its spending goes into marketing and administration.

Within the public health community, TRIPS raises concerns about access to medicines. For drugs unprotected by patent rights, because such rights are not granted, asserted or have expired, other producers can manufacture generic versions that can be sold more competitively. This leads to lower drug prices for consumers, especially important for low-income countries. However, for drugs under patent protection, producers are allowed to charge higher prices. Where a drug is needed for an important public health condition, the high cost of patented drugs becomes a particularly acute issue (WHO 2001). This tension between the economics of drug development and marketing, and the need to protect public health, came to a head in 2001 when the South African Government sought an amendment to the South African Medicines and Related Substances Control Amendment Act that would allow the import and use of cheaper generic versions of prescription drugs. This amendment was sought to allow the country to import cheaper anti-retrovirals (ARVs) to help tackle the country's HIV/AIDS epidemic. The key clause stated that the government could find and 'parallel import' the cheapest drug available, and grant 'compulsory licensing' to other companies allowing them to make copies of patented drugs without the patent holder's permission. It was argued that the rapidly rising prevalence of HIV/AIDS in the country was a public health emergency. Thirty-nine pharmaceutical companies, including GlaxoSmithKline, Merck and Roche, did not agree and launched legal action in 1998 to protect their patents.

The drug companies eventually dropped the case in April 2001 following campaigning by non-governmental organizations such as Health Action International and Médecins sans Frontières (MSF). Despite seeing the South African action as a test case to prevent other countries, such as Brazil and India, from following suit, the companies faced unexpected negative publicity and strong criticism. The clear need to further clarify the terms of the TRIPS agreement was thus recognized. In 2001, at the Ministerial Conference of the WTO held in Doha, Qatar, a Declaration on TRIPS and Public Health was agreed (known as the Doha Declaration) recognizing the right of WTO members to 'protect public health and, in particular, to promote access to medicines for all'. In addition, Paragraph 6 of the Doha Declaration instructed the TRIPS Council to address how WTO members with insufficient manufacturing capacities in pharmaceuticals can make effective use of compulsory licensing. While these countries may issue compulsory licences to import generic versions of patent-protected medicines, TRIPS rules impose constraints on the abilities of countries to authorize exports of such products. Paragraph 6 promised a solution to the export problem caused by these constraints and a further agreement to address this problem was reached in August 2003 (Correa 2004).

Despite limitations, the Doha Declaration and the TRIPS agreement provided the flexibility (strong regulations) for countries to manufacture medications or for generic medications to be exported. It allowed India – the country with the largest generic manufacturing sector – to become 'the pharmacy of the world'. However, as set out above, since the Declaration in 2001, the USA and others (including the EU) have tried, and in some cases successfully introduced, so-called 'TRIPS Plus' measures into bilateral trade agreements. One specific aspect that has been a cause of controversy in relation to the production of pharmaceuticals is the issue of *data exclusivity*. This refers to data proving the clinical efficacy and safety of a drug. Pharmaceutical companies holding patents that expire have argued that the original trial data proving the efficacy of a drug is exclusive and cannot be transferred to a generic version of such drug, which would necessitate full clinical trials to be completed at high cost and with delay. In some cases, such as the Central American Free Trade Agreement (CAFTA) countries, data exclusivity has been included in regional or bilateral trade agreements.

General Agreement on Trade in Services (GATS) and trade in health services

In the past, most services were not considered to be tradable across borders. Advances in communications technology, including the rise of e-commerce, and regulatory changes mean it is now easy and common for services to be delivered across borders. In many countries, changes in government policy have left greater room for the private sector – domestic as well as foreign – to provide services. Partly as a result of this, services have become the fastest-growing segment of the world economy, providing more than 60 per cent of global output and employment. Such changes led governments to call for the inclusion of services in trade negotiations. The result was the General Agreement on Trade in Services (GATS) agreed at the end of the Uruguay Round.

GATS defines four modes of service delivery:

• *Mode 1* – Cross-border supply, e.g. provision of diagnosis or treatment planning services in country A by suppliers in country B, via telecommunications ('telemedicine').

- *Mode 2* – Consumption abroad, e.g. movement of patients from country A to country B for treatment (medical tourism).
- *Mode 3* – Commercial presence, e.g. establishment of or investment in hospitals in country A whose owners are from country B.
- *Mode 4* – Presence of natural persons, e.g. service provision in country A by health professionals who have temporarily left country B to provide services in A (movement of health workers).

In relation to trade in health services, there has generally been growth of almost all of these modes, although there is little evidence to date that this is related directly to GATS. Some modes of trade in health services, such as the cross-border Mode 1 supply of nursing services, are unlikely to be practical. However, other services, such as processing of medical claims or transcribing medical records, can be supplied on a cross-border basis. Medical transcription services are a fast-growing industry, especially in countries with a young and highly skilled population such as India. Indian companies transcribe medical records and send the information back to American health facilities via direct satellite link. Consumption of health services abroad (Mode 2), often referred to as medical tourism, is growing, with several countries such as Thailand, Malaysia, and Singapore seeing this as an economic development opportunity. These countries aim to provide complex tertiary services at lower cost, bundle health services and then market them to foreign patients, or provide services to returning expatriates. Foreign investment in health services or 'commercial presence' (Mode 3) seeks to improve the quality of commercially available health services for those who can afford them, particularly when accompanied by new technology and know-how. This might take the form of investment in a modern hospital or health insurance management practices. The presence of natural persons (Mode 4), the least significant in total trade flows, is the most visible of the four modes. The migration of health professionals from less developed to more developed countries is the most prominent example. Bangladesh, India, Pakistan, and the Philippines, among others, are the source of large numbers of 'exported' health professionals. While evidence suggests trade in health services across all modes has increased, the effects of this on health are not well understood. The few studies that have examined the effects on countries and country health systems (e.g. Thailand, Tunisia, and the UK) have shown a mixed level of impact. For example, overall trade in health services, including export of health services, seems to provide some additional small benefit to a country's GDP. At the same time, private foreign patients may provide a lucrative source of income for the health system. Yet there is also clear evidence that in some countries foreign patients displace domestic patients or draw clinicians from the public to the private for-profit health sector.

Mode 4, the export of health professionals, has been associated with a so-called 'brain drain' in many countries. However, as foreign direct investment is increasing and a private medical sector is growing in some countries, such as, for example, India, there is evidence of health workers returning 'home' to provide services, including to medical tourists. Such an example highlights the connection between different modes of trade in health services, the complexities involved in this, and subsequent difficulty for countries to regulate or consider trade under GATS in a way that is beneficial for public health.

Finally, there are limitations to existing data on trade in services, which are not disaggregated by sector. Health services do not appear, except for health-related travel for a few countries. Some industrialized countries that do collect such data mask the information in publications to protect private businesses' confidentiality. Many countries lack data collection systems, especially as services are often provided in the private sector, with limited reporting or ability by governments to monitor volume. It is therefore difficult to discern trends in such trade, and the extent to which GATS has or will impact on them. Evidence of health services trade is limited to case studies and the effects on health systems and health outcomes are not clearly understood. There is a need for better data to track the scale and direction of trade in health services over time.

 Activity 8.3

Imagine that you needed a specialized operation but the procedure was not available in your own country. Draw up a list of some of the practical considerations you might need to take into account in seeking this treatment abroad.

Feedback

You might consider thinking about how to find a qualified practitioner, whether language would pose a barrier, how the service would be paid for, and what recourse you would have if the operation was performed incorrectly.

Regulatory capacity and coordination to manage risks associated with trade agreements

Trade agreements lead, at least in theory, to substantial benefits – economic growth, lower cost, and wider access to goods through trade barrier reductions; and through involvement in trading blocs, the protection of nations from others' power. But the trade regime itself, because of its increasingly interventionist nature, is a growing source of risk. This risk requires management, and this is the role of regulation. Thus, the trade regime is contributing to regulatory demand, ironic given the purpose of trade is usually about increasing freedom of the market, and is placing enormous strains on the capacities of states to regulate.

The regulatory capacity requisite for appropriate negotiation, monitoring, and management of trade agreements is expensive, skill-intensive, and requires considerable infrastructure. This capacity to manage trade agreements varies markedly between countries, with small and particularly poorer states at a considerable disadvantage. Trade agreements challenge the capacity of developed states to regulate activities that extend beyond their borders. Many developing states lack even the capacity to regulate domestically.

Once a country signs onto intellectual property standards, for example, it needs patent offices, and scientific capacity to evaluate pharmaceutical patents. Most developing countries simply lack this capacity. Additionally, there is the issue that even for large developing countries, signing up to international intellectual property standards and setting up patent offices may not actually serve to support their development interests. It is a country's national development objectives that should drive their intellectual property strategy.

Despite pressure from developed countries for developing countries to view patenting as key to technological development and to conform to the former's patent law standards, some emerging markets, notably the BRICS countries (Brazil, Russia, India, China, and South Africa), have begun to develop alternative regulation that better suits their own unique environments and interests. Such alternatives may better maintain domestic policy-making space and allow priority to be placed on addressing social goals within the patent context, such as by using compulsory licensing to provide access to medicines.

Significantly, none of the BRICS countries are part of the TPP negotiations, with their TRIPS Plus standards a core objective.

Summary

The WTO is one of the institutional pillars of economic globalization, but international trade influence is increasingly channelled through other mechanisms. The trade liberalization mediated by trade agreements used to be about removing tariff barriers to trade, but since the Uruguay Round especially, trade agreements have also addressed non-tariff barriers, areas not formerly part of the trade regime. The various trade agreements established influence both the broad determinants of health, as well as the nature of health services and financing, in all countries. Thus, management of the risks and harnessing the opportunities associated with trade agreements requires significant regulatory capacity and coordination – something that needs significant capacity-building efforts in many countries. The extent to which trade regulation shapes availability, access, and price of pharmaceuticals is further explored in the next chapter.

References

Blouin, C., Drager, N. and Smith, R. (eds) (2006) *International Trade in Health Services and the GATS: Current Issues and Debates*. Washington, DC: World Bank.

Correa, C. (2004) *Implementation of the WTO General Council Decision on Para 6 of the Doha Declaration on the TRIPS Agreement and Public Health*. EDM Series No. 16. Geneva: World Health Organization.

Fidler, D.P., Drager, N. and Lee, K. (2009) Managing the pursuit of health and wealth: the key challenges, *The Lancet*, 373 (9660): 325–31.

Light, D.W. and Warburton, R. (2011) Demythologizing the high costs of pharmaceutical research, *BioSocieties*, 6(1): 34–50.

Smith, R., Lee, K. and Drager, N. (2009a) Trade and health: an agenda for action, *The Lancet*, 373 (9665): 768–73.

Smith, R.D., Chanda, R. and Tangcharoensathien, V. (2009b) Trade in health-related services, *The Lancet*, 373 (9663): 593–601.

Trading Economics (2013) Tariff rate; applied; simple mean; all products (%) in world. [http://www.tradingeconomics.com/world/tariff-rate-applied-simple-mean-all-products-percent-wb-data.html].

WHO (2001) *Globalization, TRIPS and Access to Pharmaceuticals*. WHO Policy Perspectives on Medicines No. 3, March. Geneva: World Health Organization.

WHO (2002) *Public Health Implications of the WTO Multilateral Trade Agreements*, WHO Training Course. Geneva: World Health Organization.

WHO/WTO (2002) *WTO Agreements and Public Health*. Geneva: World Trade Organization and World Health Organization [http://www.wto.org/english/res_e/booksp_e/who_wto_e.pdf].

WTO (2001) *European Communities: Measures Affecting Asbestos and Asbestos-Containing Products*. Report of the Appellate Body, 12 March. Geneva: World Trade Organization. [www.wto.org].

WTO (2003) *TRIPS and Pharmaceutical Patents*. Fact Sheet. Geneva: World Trade Organization.

WTO (2013) *Welcome to the Regional Trade Agreements Information System (RTA-IS)*. Geneva: World Trade Organization [http://rtais.wto.org/UI/PublicAllRTAList.aspx].

Globalization, commercialization, and the tobacco and alcohol sectors

Benjamin Hawkins and Jeff Collin

Overview

In this chapter, you will learn about the changing structure of the tobacco and alcohol industries over recent decades, which will provide valuable insights into the relationship between global change and health. Developments in the international trade regime have led to an increasing concentration of ownership of these industries among a small number of multinational corporations. This, in turn, has had a significant impact on rates of consumption and harm, also evidenced in the global rise in non-communicable diseases further discussed in Chapter 11, with both industries reorienting their strategies towards markets in low- and middle-income countries. In this context, traditional forms of health governance are incapable of effectively responding to the threat posed by tobacco and alcohol. The need for global solutions to a global pandemic has given rise to a unique policy initiative: the WHO's Framework Convention on Tobacco Control. However, no equivalent framework convention exists for alcohol control policies. Instead, alcohol policy at the global level is set out in the World Health Organization's *Global Strategy to Reduce the Harmful Use of Alcohol* (WHO 2010), a looser document lacking the legal force of the frameworks convention.

Learning objectives

After working through this chapter, you will be able to:

- compare the threats to global health posed by transnational tobacco and alcohol companies
- describe the impact of trade liberalization on the development of the global tobacco and alcohol industries
- explain the emergence of the WHO's Framework Convention on Tobacco Control, and the absence of a similar framework for alcohol
- evaluate the opportunities and threats for effective health policies posed by processes of globalization and commercialization

Key terms

Pandemic: A pandemic is where a disease has extensively and widely spread on a scale that crosses international boundaries, usually affecting a large number of people.

Smoking prevalence: The percentage of a given population that currently smokes tobacco.

> **Trade liberalization:** The process by which national economies become more open to cross-border flows of goods, services, and capital.

Tobacco, alcohol, and global health

Consumption of cigarettes and other tobacco products and exposure to tobacco smoke collectively constitute the world's leading preventable cause of deaths in adults. Responsible for around one in ten of all adult deaths, smoking-attributable deaths are projected to rise to 8.3 million annually by 2030 (Levy et al. 2013). The global scale of tobacco's health impacts merits the use of the term pandemic, and this pandemic is undergoing rapid acceleration. Mortality levels attributable to tobacco have increased by about 45 per cent since 1990, and are expected to double to around 10 million per annum (or one in six adult deaths) by 2030 unless widespread and effective interventions are rapidly implemented.

According to the WHO, alcohol is the world's third largest risk factor for disease burden after tobacco and hypertension, responsible for around 2.25 million deaths per year (WHO 2011). In the Western Pacific and the Americas, it is the leading risk factor and in Europe it is the second largest. Alcohol is also one of the leading causes of death within the 18–25 year age group (Jones et al. 2008). In Russia, alcohol use was responsible for more than half of all deaths among men aged 15–54 (Zaridze et al. 2009). Recent decades have seen an increase in alcohol consumption in many countries, associated with increased affordability. In the UK, for example, alcohol is now 61 per cent more affordable in 2012 than in 1980 as a result of rising incomes, which have outstripped rises in prices (HSCIC 2013). This overall trend has coincided with increases in consumption by females in many countries, with noticeable consequences for rates of alcohol-related harm among women.

While there are clear similarities between the health burden of tobacco and alcohol, there are important differences in the type of harms associated with each. Tobacco and alcohol use are associated with a range of chronic diseases, and because of the impairment of the senses brought about by alcohol consumption, it is an increased risk factor for accidents and road deaths (e.g. through drink driving). In addition, while there is no safe level of tobacco use, alcohol may be consumed safely at low levels, As such, we need to apply slightly different lenses when considering the health impact of alcohol versus tobacco. As many people underestimate consumption and overestimate the amount they can consume safely, public health messages about healthy drinking patterns are highly problematic.

Tobacco industry actors are singled out for special treatment and largely excluded from policy-making at the country and global levels. The pariah status of the tobacco industry is in part a result of the level of knowledge we have about their activities through the release of internal industry documents following litigation in the USA in the 1990s (Hurt et al. 2009). Much of the academic literature and the policy discourse surrounding tobacco control treats the product and the industry that produces it as a special case, given the uniquely harmful nature of tobacco and the often underhand tactics employed by the tobacco industry to defend their interests (Casswell 2013). For example, the political declaration of the UN High Meeting on the Prevention and Control of Non-communicable Diseases precluded engagement with the tobacco industry while welcoming partnerships with other industry actors, including the food and alcohol industries (WHO 2012). While in no means underplaying the harmful nature of smoking and the mendacity of the tobacco industry, this chapter seeks to problematize tobacco 'exceptionalism'. It argues that we should extend the same level of scrutiny to corporate actors in other industries that produce harmful products, such as alcohol. There are similarities in strategies between the two industries.

Global health issues

The global distribution of tobacco consumption is undergoing rapid change, and its diverse social, economic, and health impacts are becoming increasingly inequitable. A broad decline in smoking prevalence across most high-income countries in recent decades has coincided with substantial increases among low- and middle-income countries. Given the lengthy delay between the onset of smoking and tobacco's health impacts, this global shift is being slowly but inexorably followed by a redistribution of tobacco-related disease and death.

- About half of all tobacco-related deaths now occur in low- and middle-income countries.
- By 2030, low- and middle-income countries will account for around 70 per cent of all tobacco-related deaths.
- In China, annual tobacco deaths are expected to reach 2 million by 2025.
- In India, around 80 million males under the age of 35 will eventually be killed by tobacco (Thun and da Costa e Silva 2003).

Within this overall shift in the tobacco pandemic there predictably exists enormous diversity among low- and middle-income countries, and the pandemic remains strongly differentiated by, *inter alia*, region and gender, with rates of smoking by males outstripping those of women.

Though national patterns of tobacco consumption and its health impacts continue to differ widely, they can be considered to be following broadly comparable trajectories. A four-stage model developed for WHO (Lopez et al. 1994) offers a conceptual framework within which the evolution of national epidemics can be related to the broader pandemic (Figure 9.1). The key characteristics of each stage can be summarized as follows:

- *Stage 1* – low prevalence of cigarette smoking at under 20 per cent, largely confined to males, while rates of lung cancer or other chronic diseases caused by smoking have not yet demonstrably increased.
- *Stage 2* – prevalence of smoking among men exceeds 50 per cent, evidence of increases among women, younger age of take-up, and an increasing burden of tobacco-related disease among men.
- *Stage 3* – convergence of prevalence of smoking by males and females given a clear reduction among men and a more gradual decline among women, but the long time lag in tobacco's health impacts result in smoking-attributable mortality reaching 10–30 per cent of all deaths.
- *Stage 4* – marked reduction in smoking prevalence of both males and females, and smoking-attributable deaths peak at 30–35 per cent among men before declining, while such deaths rise to 20–25 per cent of all deaths among women.

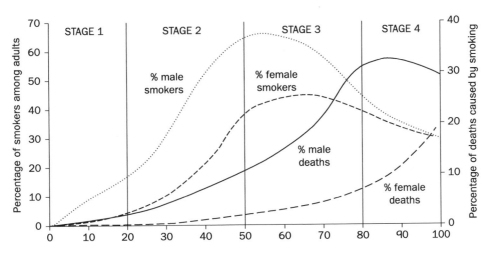

Figure 9.1 Four stages of the tobacco epidemic

Source: Thun and da Costa e Silva (2003)

✏ **Activity 9.1**

On the basis of the WHO model described above and depicted in Figure 9.1, try to allocate your country or region to one of the four stages of the tobacco epidemic. Explain why you placed it in that stage and give examples to support your decision.

Feedback

Sub-Saharan Africa is the region that most clearly exhibits the attributes of Stage 1; China, Japan, Southeast Asia, Latin America, and North Africa broadly fit with Stage 2; Eastern Europe and Southern Europe can be characterized as being in Stage 3; Western Europe, the USA, Canada, and Australia can be identified among those countries in Stage 4.

While tobacco clearly constitutes a global health problem, this exercise demonstrates the diversity that continues to characterize national experiences of the pandemic. Such diversity has important implications for the future development of the tobacco industry, as the evolution of national epidemics is shaped by tobacco companies and impacts on their profitability. You should consider such implications as you progress through the remainder of this chapter.

As with tobacco, alcohol-related harms are not limited to the developed world, but increasingly affect low- and middle-income countries. Low- and middle-income countries are now experiencing significant and increasing rates of alcohol-related harm, associated with rising consumption and a shift to 'ern' drinking patterns. As with tobacco, though, these overall trends mask wide variations between countries. Much of the world's population is, for example, teetotal (often for religious or cultural reasons) and patterns of consumption among those who do drink vary widely, often, but not exclusively, by gender. Like non-commercial forms of tobacco use, much of the alcohol consumed in certain parts of the world, such as Sub-Saharan Africa, is home brew or moonshine products, produced and sold unofficially. What unites the health threat posed by alcohol and tobacco is the extent to which both products are being marketed in populous low- and middle-income country markets by large transnational corporations. As with the entry of transnational tobacco corporations into new markets, transnational alcohol corporations adopt branding, marketing, and pricing strategies that drive overall consumption and harm.

Globalization and transnational tobacco corporations

While the geographical scope of tobacco use has long been extensive, the contemporary scale of its mass use, and related health impacts, are much more recent. The current pandemic represents the outcome of the huge changes arising from the development of automated cigarette rolling machines in the late nineteenth century and driven forward by the largest transnational tobacco corporations (TTCs). Key to this strategy was the development of the white stick cigarette as the standard product marketed across the globe, and the application of branding and advertising strategies to drive sales and consumption. The cigarette was to become established as arguably the most successful commercial product of the twentieth century. Importantly for global health, however, it appears that the commercial potential of the cigarette has not yet been fully realized.

Key features of the global political economy have already effected a transformation in the structure and prospects of the tobacco industry, creating enormous commercial opportunities while exacerbating impacts on global health. The years since 1990 have seen an increasingly inequitable burden of tobacco consumption. This is due to the recent global expansion of a handful of TTCs – including Philip Morris, British American Tobacco, Japan Tobacco International – that are now clearly established as the primary vectors of the tobacco pandemic.

From a global health perspective, it is important to note that trade liberalization has inequitable impacts, leading to:

• an overall increase in tobacco consumption globally and within low- and middle-income countries;
• a large and significant impact on smoking in low-income countries;
• a significant, if smaller, impact on middle-income countries;
• no substantive impact on tobacco consumption in higher-income countries.

Transnational tobacco corporations' traditional sources of profit in the markets of North America and Western Europe have begun to be eroded in recent decades from the combined threats of regulation, declining consumption, and litigation. Developments in the global political economy have, however, created substantial new opportunities in what TTCs refer to as emerging markets. Among key drivers of recent global expansion are the following:

• formation of the World Trade Organization (WTO), including the Trade Related Aspects of Intellectual Property (TRIPS) agreement on intellectual property rights and the creation of a dispute resolution mechanism;
• increasing prevalence of regional trade agreements and bilateral investment treaties between states, many of which include 'investor state agreements' under which corporations can sue state governments for infringements of their commercial rights and freedoms;

- the decline and privatization of previously state-owned tobacco monopolies, encouraged by the International Monetary Fund;
- increased integration of large markets in low- and middle-income countries with the global economy.

Transnational tobacco corporations quickly recognized the opportunities inherent in such changes, using the General Agreement on Tariffs and Trade (GATT) treaties, the predecessor to the WTO, to challenge government monopolies and to gain market access to South East Asian markets including Thailand in the 1980s (Chantornvong and McCargo 2001). More recently, TTCs have used WTO agreements and bilateral investment treaties to challenge the Australian Government's decision to introduce plain packaging for cigarettes. The measures under which all tobacco products will be sold in identical packets with product names stated in a uniform font and typeface are, according to TTCs, both trade restrictive and an affront to their property right, including the freedom to use their trademarks as they see fit.

In March 2012, Ukraine initiated dispute proceedings with the WTO claiming that the legislation violated several WTO agreements, including the GATT, the Agreement on the Application of Sanitary and Phytosanitary Measures (SPS), and the Agreement on Technical Barriers to Trade (TBT). Subsequently, Honduras and Uruguay have filed similar complaints under the WTO dispute resolution mechanism. British American Tobacco (BAT) is paying legal expenses for Ukraine and Honduras, while Philip Morris International is doing the same for the Dominican Republic. In this case, as in that of Thailand, health objectives and trade objectives potentially come into conflict, creating powerful arguments for tobacco to be explicitly excluded from future global, regional, and bilateral trade agreements.

✎ Activity 9.2

Given the precedent of the Thailand GATT case, and based on what you have learned about WTO agreements, briefly identify ways in which the following health measures might conflict with the Technical Barriers to Trade (TBT), the General Agreement on Trade in Services (GATS), and the TRIPS agreements:

1 Prohibiting 'misleading descriptors' on tobacco products (i.e. use of terms like 'light' and 'mild', which have been perceived as suggesting reduced risk).
2 Requiring full public disclosure of ingredients, additives, and flavourings for each cigarette brand.
3 Plain packaging of tobacco products, which requires all brands to be sold in identical packaging with enlarged graphic health warnings that make health impacts more prominent while reducing the visual appeal of the brand.
4 Fully comprehensive advertising bans that cover brand sharing (developing alternative products bearing the name of tobacco advertising), sponsorships and point of sale promotions (in-store displays), in addition to traditional forms of advertising (e.g. cinema, radio, television, and newspaper advertisements).

Feedback

1 This could be viewed as a violation of company trademarks. Japan has repeatedly threatened to challenge a European Union directive prohibiting such terminology

(Mild Seven is a key international brand for JTI). Such a measure could conceivably be viewed as infringing either the TBT or TRIPS agreements.

2 Compulsory ingredient disclosure could impinge on the protections to product information offered by TRIPS. Yet such measures are increasingly viewed as important both in enabling consumers to make informed decisions and in allowing the future development of more effective means of regulating the composition of such harmful products.

3 Stringent requirements on packaging and labelling could be interpreted as incompatible with the protections offered by the TRIPS and TBT agreements. Trademarks such as those on packs can be considered a form of intellectual property and denying companies the right to use these trademarks may infringe their intellectual property rights, thus creating barriers to commerce.

4 While the GATT arbitration panel upheld Thai legislation, it has been argued that a different verdict might now be reached under GATS, particularly in a case where such fully comprehensive prohibitions were envisaged.

Such interpretations should be viewed with caution in the absence of clear precedents. It does, however, seem reasonable to expect that at least some of these tensions are likely to be explored in the near future. The Thai case is particularly instructive since it serves to demonstrate how trade agreements can mitigate against measures that might reasonably be viewed as protecting health, while also highlighting the substantial scope remaining for effective regulation.

Transnational alcohol corporations

Where the tobacco industry has led, the alcohol industry has followed. Economic liberalization at the global level has facilitated similar growth and consolidation within the alcohol industry. Production of alcoholic beverages is concentrated among a small number of large transnational corporations. Unlike the tobacco industry, which has focused on the sale and marketing of a single dominant product, the white stick cigarette, the alcohol market consists of a number of different drinks categories with different corporations active within and between these sectors, as evident in a review of the largest companies. Table 9.1 lists the largest companies in each product category. Consolidation of ownership has been particularly marked in the beer and spirits markets, although there is evidence of consolidation in the wine market and the emergence of global wine brands:

- The 26 largest alcohol corporations had a turnover of $155 billion in 2005, generating profits of $26 billion.
- Alcohol companies are among the most profitable in the world, surpassed only by tobacco companies (Gilmore et al. 2010).
- The 10 largest alcohol corporations (all of which are beer producers) accounted for 48 per cent of global alcohol sales by volume in 2005.
- By 2006, the world's four largest beer producers controlled 45.5 per cent of the global market, up from 14.9 per cent in 1980.
- In 2006, the five largest spirit producers controlled 46.6 per cent of the market globally, compared with 32.4 per cent in 1991.
- In some Latin American countries, single producers control over 95 per cent of the domestic beer markets (Jernigan 2009).

Table 9.1 The five largest global alcohol producers by sector

Beer	Spirits	Wine
InBev	Diageo	Constellation Brands
SABMiller	Pernod Ricard	E&J Gallo Winery
Anheuser-Busch	United Spirits	The Wine Group
Heineken	Bacardi	The Foster's Wine Estate
Carlsberg Breweries	Beam Global Spirits	Pernod Ricard

Source: Jernigan (2009).

Concentration of ownership has increased competition and led to an increasing reliance by producers on marketing and promotional activity. This is particularly the case in mature markets such as the UK and the USA, where increased competition has led to a reduction in prices, encouraging corporations to pursue greater sales volumes to protect their profits. Similarly, the dominant position enjoyed by some producers in developing markets can lead to monopoly pricing and results in significant marketing activities (Jernigan 2009).

Given the powerful position of the largest TACs, the size of these markets and their relatively weak regulatory frameworks, emerging markets offer the possibility of significant profits for TACs. As such, their strategic focus is shifting to these and, as with tobacco, international trade law is playing a crucial role in this process. The desire for market access and favourable regulatory environments in these countries is at least in part responsible for the opposition by spirit producers to a new law to introduce a minimum unit price for alcohol in the UK (Holden and Hawkins 2013). This policy undermines self-regulatory approaches promoted by the industry in both traditional and developing markets. Having failed to prevent the law through lobbying and other activities, the policy has been challenged by the industry under EU trade law.

Developing global brands

Premium international brands constitute the fastest growing portion of the world cigarette market with annual sales growing at about 5 per cent during the 1990s. They are of key strategic significance to TTCs since they offer higher prices, production volumes, economies of scale and, crucially, opportunities to coherently build perceptions of a brand on a cross-national basis. For BAT:

> International brands are defined as those brands that are available in a number of markets and currently sell, or have the potential to sell, significant volumes in the future. They are generally priced at a higher or premium level, have consistent pack designs and communications to the smoker with a clear target consumer in mind . . . The fact that a 'foreign' brand is sold on another market is not sufficient to justify its description as an International Brand, because the latter involves a mix of global availability, plus perception of internationality to the consumer.
>
> (BATCo 1994)

The template for this strategy was set by Philip Morris's success in transforming Marlboro from a stagnant American brand in the early 1960s, to a business phenomenon and one of the few truly global brands. Marlboro continues to dwarf its competitors, accounting for 8.4 per cent of global cigarette consumption, a success that is inseparable from the brilliance and ubiquity of its advertising and marketing. The Marlboro Man was declared by *Advertising Age* to be the number one advertising icon of the twentieth century, and the campaign transformed the fortunes of the brand. It established a strong image that has been applied consistently across markets, with minor adaptations to accommodate local norms.

Similar use of branding and advertising has been made by TACs to create global brands in the beer, spirits, cider, and latterly wine markets. These are often offered alongside 'local' brands in each market, which are nevertheless owned, controlled or distributed and marketed by the TACs. This has been most widely documented in mature markets such as the UK and the USA. As TACs increasingly focus their strategies on emerging markets, they are promoting global brands and local consumer products as safer alternatives to homebrew.

✎ **Activity 9.3**

The diverse promotional activities undertaken by tobacco and alcohol companies are directed at differing audiences and, in combination, pursue multiple objectives. Make a brief list of the strategic advantages that might be offered by:

1 An international sport sponsorship, such as the football World Cup, Olympics or Formula One motor racing.
2 A campaign to eliminate the use of child labour in tobacco production.
3 A campaign by a brewer active in low-income countries to improve water supply and sanitation.

Give attention to the regulatory environment in which tobacco companies have to operate, where conventional forms of advertising are increasingly denied to them.

Feedback

1 Sports sponsorship has assumed increasing importance as advertising restrictions have been tightened, serving to maintain a television presence for cigarette brands. International sponsorships can also serve to promote the global expansion of a brand. Sponsorship can also exert political influence both via the creation of influential allies (e.g. sports organizations and ruling bodies) and opportunities for corporate hospitality with key regulators. While tobacco advertising is excluded from the football World Cup and Olympics, alcohol brands are key partners for both events, giving them significant influence and marketing exposure.
2 The Elimination of Child Labour in Tobacco Growing Foundation was formed in 2001. BAT was instrumental in its formation, and the world's leading cigarette manufacturers and tobacco leaf companies are now members. The need to rebuild their reputations to secure their long-term investment and reduce the political pressure for legislation explains why tobacco companies have embraced corporate social

responsibility. The interest in eliminating child labour is strategically well chosen, since it appears to demonstrate a responsible commitment to the well-being of the societies in which TTCs operate, and therefore might serve to reduce criticism and calls for regulation.

3 Brewer SABMiller has focused attention on the issue of water supply and sanitation through its campaigns, website, and social media outlets. Arguably a campaign of this nature reflects both the severity of the issue of water supply facing the continent and its roots in South Africa. Focusing on issues such as water supply diverts attention away from the harms associated with alcohol and positions SABMiller as part of the solution to social problems, rather than a cause.

Negotiating the Framework Convention on Tobacco Control

A text laboriously developed following two preliminary meetings of a working group and across six sessions of an Inter-governmental Negotiating Body (INB) received the unanimous endorsement of the 56th World Health Assembly in May 2003. This concluded four years of negotiations for a Framework Convention on Tobacco Control (FCTC), WHO's first attempt to exercise its constitutional authority to develop a global public health treaty. Based on recognition of the challenges posed by globalization, the FCTC is intended to create an international public health movement capable both of addressing transnational issues and of providing a powerful resource in support of national health efforts. Among the key features of the final text are provisions encouraging countries to do the following:

- enact comprehensive bans on tobacco advertising, promotion, and sponsorship;
- require large rotating health warnings on packaging, to cover at least 30 per cent of principal display areas, and with provision for pictorial warnings;
- prohibit the use of misleading descriptors such as 'light' or 'mild';
- increase taxation of tobacco products;
- provide greater protection from involuntary exposure to tobacco smoke;
- develop measures to combat smuggling.

The FCTC text failed to include language that would clarify its status in relationship to existing trade agreements ('health vs. trade' being the single most divisive issue during negotiations) and is lacking in binding obligations, although these may be developed further by a number of issue-specific protocols. However, progress on developing these protocols has been slow. This reflects the enormous complexity of drafting regulations that suit such a wide array of countries, and their differing political priorities. The first protocol to be developed focused on illicit trade, an area both of great political and economic concern and which it was believed held the most common ground for action among governments. Despite evidence that TTCs had supported smuggling in the past, their formal position was now to support strong anti-smuggling measures. In 2013, the protocol on illicit trade was opened for signature by contracting parties to the FCTC and remained open until January 2014. Subsequently, the protocol will need to be ratified by national governments and legislatures.

Such caveats notwithstanding, however, the final text of the FCTC was a remarkable advance on the heavily criticized preceding draft and was broadly welcomed by health groups. The significance of the FCTC, however, arguably resides primarily in the process of its development rather than in the content of the text.

Corporate documents from BAT also indicate the scale of industry efforts to influence the negotiation process. An internal document from BAT described the FCTC as 'an unprecedented challenge to the tobacco industry's freedom to continue doing business', accepted that an agreement was likely, and established a strategy for minimizing its potential impact. Seeking to build support among potentially sympathetic states, health and finance ministers were to be targeted as 'our priority stakeholders', while growers, unions, and trade organizations were also identified as potentially useful. The document claimed 'some success at governmental level' in stimulating favourable contributions to the drafting process by Brazil, China, Germany, Argentina, and Zimbabwe (BAT Indonesia n.d.). Additionally, tobacco companies were sporadically successful in ensuring that their representatives formed part of negotiating delegations.

The FCTC process also entailed efforts to include civil society, efforts that were necessarily partial and a predictable source of tension within a fundamentally essentially state-centric policy process. The terms of participation of non-governmental organizations (NGOs) remained strongly contested throughout the negotiation process.

The involvement of civil society organizations in the FCTC process was greatly enhanced by the formation and development of the Framework Convention Alliance (FCA). At the two working group meetings that preceded the formal negotiations of the INB, civil society participation had been largely confined to high-income country NGOs and international health-based NGOs. By February 2003, the FCA encompassed more than 180 NGOs from over 70 countries, and had established itself as an important lobbying alliance. Coordinated via the FCA, NGOs in official relations with WHO were able to exploit their limited access to fulfil significant lobbying, educational, and monitoring roles. The expertise accumulated within the FCA became a key resource, particularly in progressive alliance with the African and South-East Asian regions. Additionally, a few prominent advocates were occasionally included within the official delegations of member states.

The impact of civil society in the final negotiations was significantly hampered by increasing unease among member states opposed to a powerful text. The designation of most negotiating sessions of the final INB as informal provided a simple mechanism for the exclusion of NGO participants; a reduction of access and transparency reportedly supported by delegations including the USA and China.

✏ Activity 9.4

How significant is the Framework Convention on Tobacco Control as an innovation in global health governance? Write two paragraphs explaining its importance. In your answer, consider the potential impact of the FCTC on other areas such as alcohol and food policies.

Feedback

The Convention is widely regarded as a comparatively impressive document, incorporating more substantial commitments than many anticipated. Its impact on health will, however, be dependent on widespread adoption by states, effective implementation at national level, and on whether there exists the political will for the further negotiation of protocols (requiring more specific obligations). Of greater significance than the FCTC itself, however, are likely to be the multiple and diverse impacts of the process of its negotiation. As an innovation in global health governance, it represents a partial opening to non-state actors. Civil society groups played important roles but their participation was circumscribed, while the official involvement of TTCs in the process was restricted to the public hearings.

Beyond its significance as a tobacco control measure, the FCTC assumes broader relevance as a response to the restricted capacity of national governance to effectively address global health risks. It can also be viewed as a unique effort to regulate the conduct of transnational corporations. It is clear that the FCTC marks tobacco control policy out from other issues at the global level. There is no equivalent to the FCTC for alcohol or food regulation despite the harms associated with drinking and unhealthy diets. Perhaps the FCTC offers a model for regulation in these areas too. It is a clear example for campaigners seeking stronger regulation of alcohol and tobacco at the global level to point to as an example to follow in these areas. At the same time, industry actors seek to underline the differences between tobacco and other products. Much will depend on the success of the FCTC going forwards and the ability of governments to draft, ratify, and enforce subsequent protocols.

Summary

In this chapter, we have examined the similarities between the globalization of the tobacco and alcohol industries and the consequences this globalization has for public health. Both these industries have used trade liberalization as a means of expanding their reach beyond traditional markets in Europe and North America to emerging markets in low- and middle-income countries. Through the creation of global brands and marketing strategies, this process has driven consumption leading to significant current and future health problems for populous countries with limited finances and health systems resources. The global nature of these industries necessitates global policy solutions. We have seen how the FCTC stands as a demonstration of a countervailing force to the tobacco industry. Despite the level of harm caused by alcohol, and the similarities which exist between both the alcohol and tobacco industries and the types of intervention that may be developed to counter tobacco- and alcohol-related mortality and morbidity, no similar convention has yet been adopted for alcohol.

References

BAT Indonesia (n.d.) *A Study on the Smokers of International Brands*. Guildford Depository, Bates No. 400458935–9056.

BATCo Marketing Intelligence Department (1994) *International Brands 1988–1992*. Guildford Depository, January, Bates No. 500056134–6179.

Casswell, S. (2013) Vested interests in addiction research and policy: why do we not see the corporate interests of the alcohol industry as clearly as we see those of the tobacco industry?, *Addiction*, 108: 680–5.

Chantornvong, S. and McCargo, D. (2001) Political economy of tobacco control in Thailand, *Tobacco Control*, 10: 48–54.

Gilmore, A.B., Branston, J.R. and Sweanor, D. (2010) The case for OFSMOKE: how tobacco price regulation is needed to promote the health of markets, government revenue and the public, *Tobacco Control*, 19: 423–30.

Holden, C. and Hawkins, B. (2013) 'Whisky gloss': the alcohol industry, devolution and policy communities in Scotland, *Public Policy and Administration*, 28 (3): 253–73.

HSCIC (2013) *Statistics on Alcohol – England, 2013*, May, p. 17. Leeds: Health and Social Care Information Centre [http://www.hscic.gov.uk/catalogue/PUB10932].

Hurt, R.D., Ebbert, J.O., Muggli, M.E., Lockhart, N.J. and Robertson, C.R. (2009) Open doorway to truth: legacy of the Minnesota tobacco trial, *Mayo Clinic Proceedings*, 84 (5): 446–56.

Jernigan, D. (2009) The global alcohol industry: an overview, *Addiction*, 104 (suppl. 1): 6–12.

Jones, L., Bellis, M.A., Dedman, D., Sumnall, H. and Tocque, K. (2008) Alcohol-attributable fractions for England: alcohol-attributable mortality and hospital admissions. Liverpool: Centre for Public Health, Liverpool John Moores University and North West Public Health Observatory [http://www.alcohollearning centre.org.uk/_library/AlcoholAttributableFractions.pdf].

Levy, D., Ellis, J., Mays, D. and Huang, A.-T. (2013) Smoking-related deaths averted due to three years of policy progress, *Bulletin of the World Health Organization*, 91: 509–18.

Lopez, A., Collishaw, N. and Piha, T. (1994) A descriptive model of the cigarette epidemic in developed countries, *Tobacco Control*, 3: 242–7.

Thun, M. and da Costa e Silva, V.L. (2003) Introduction and overview of global tobacco surveillance, in O. Shafey, S. Dolwick and G.E. Guindon (eds) *Tobacco Control Country Profiles* (2nd edn). Atlanta, GA: American Cancer Society.

WHO (2010) *Global Strategy to Reduce the Harmful Use of Alcohol*. Geneva: World Health Organization.

WHO (2011) *Global Status Report on Alcohol and Health*. Geneva: World Health Organization.

WHO (2012) *Political Declaration of the High-level Meeting of the General Assembly on the Prevention and Control of Non-communicable Diseases* [http://www.who.int/nmh/events/un_ncd_summit2011/political_declaration_en.pdf, accessed 20 March 2014].

Zaridze, D., Brennan, P., Boreham, J., Boroda, A., Karpov, R., Lazarev, A. et al. (2009) Alcohol and cause-specific mortality in Russia: a retrospective case-control study of 48,557 adult deaths, *The Lancet*, 373 (9682): 2201–14.

The globalization of the pharmaceutical industry

10

Joan Busfield

Overview

This chapter examines the structure of the pharmaceutical industry, the consolidation of top companies over recent decades, and the particular importance of western companies and markets. It looks at patented drugs and market bestsellers, at generic drugs, and at research and development in the industry. It then considers the extent of the industry's power and the extent to which it is becoming globalized. It examines the agencies that regulate the industry and the adequacy of the drug approval process. Finally, it explores the consequences of a globalizing pharmaceutical industry.

Learning objectives

After working through this chapter, you will be able to:

- describe the changing structure of the pharmaceutical industry and the extent to which it is becoming globalized
- identify the sources of the pharmaceutical industry's power
- understand the mechanisms used to regulate the industry, particularly product approval
- outline the commercial biases of the pharmaceutical industry and their consequences

Key terms

Drug approval agencies: National and international bodies that must approve a drug before it can be released onto the market.

Generic drug: A copy of a medicine produced once its patent ends, usually sold under its chemical not brand name.

Medicalization: The transformation of social and personal problems into ones held to require medical intervention.

Multinational company: A company whose manufacturing, research and development, and sales activities are spread across many countries.

Patent: A formal licence that an invention cannot be copied in the jurisdiction for which it is applied.

Regulatory capture: The process by which an independent regulatory agency takes on the values and interests of the group whose activities it regulates.

How is the pharmaceutical industry structured?

The pharmaceutical industry is a major industry in the global economy whose worldwide sales amounted to around US$950 billion in 2013 (IMS Health 2013), more than the gross national product of many low-income countries. The market is dominated by a small number of large multinational companies (see Table 10.1), with nine of the top ten having head offices in the USA or Europe (Teva, a recent entrant, has headquarters in Israel). These companies have mostly used mergers and acquisitions as the means to increase their size, but over the longer term their share of the global market has not increased. The spate of mergers in the 1990s increased the top ten companies' share from roughly one-third of world revenue (Tarabusi and Vickery 1998) to nearly a half in 2003 (Busfield 2003). However, while mergers and acquisitions have continued, the top ten's proportion of the total market has declined to around one-third as companies in China, India, and Brazil have expanded their sales volume (IMS Health 2013).

The US company Pfizer was the leading pharmaceutical company in the world by sales value throughout most of the first decade of this century, achieving its position as market leader after acquiring Warner-Lambert in 2000 and Pharmacia in 2003. Pharmacia had European origins, created by a merger between the Swedish company Kabi Vitrum and the Italian Carlo Erba in 1993. The Swiss company Novartis, the current market leader, resulted from a merger between two Swiss companies, Ciba-Geigy and Sandoz in 1996. Then in 2009 it acquired Alcon, a leading company in eye-care products. The dominance of western companies in the top ten is unsurprising given that North America and Europe account for around 60 per cent of world revenues in pharmaceuticals (see Table 10.2). The USA is the largest market with around 30 per cent by sales value, followed by Japan with around 12 per cent.

Leading pharmaceutical companies are among the largest companies in the world in terms of revenues and many are highly profitable. Their profits come largely from the sale of patented drugs. A patent is the assertion of ownership over an innovation or idea, known as an intellectual property right (IPR). This right can be claimed if an invention is new, involves an 'inventive step', and is capable of industrial application. The standard length of a patent is twenty years, though there are various means for extending this,

Table 10.1 Top ten pharmaceutical companies by sales value, 2012

Corporation	Rank	Headquarters	Sales value (US$ million)
Novartis	1	Switzerland	50,761
Pfizer	2	USA	46,930
Merck & Co.	3	USA	40,115
Sanofi	4	France	37,780
Roche	5	Switzerland	35,069
GlaxoSmithKline	6	UK	32,714
AstraZeneca	7	UK	31,893
Johnson & Johnson	8	USA	27,933
Abbott	9	USA	26,715
Teva	10	Israel	24,846

Source: IMS Health (2013).

Table 10.2 World pharmaceutical sales revenues* by region, 2003

World market	Sales 2012 (US$ billion)	%
North America	349.0	36.4
Europe (EU + non-EU)	224.3	23.4
Asia, Africa and Australia	168.3	17.5
Japan	112.1	11.7
Latin America	68.6	7.2
Total	959.0	100

*Sales include prescription and certain over-the-counter sales.
Source: IMS Health (2013).

including by making small changes to a product or process. A drug company usually seeks a patent once a new substance with therapeutic potential is identified in order to secure exclusive rights over its production and commercial use. This allows the company to set a (higher) price commensurate with this exclusivity once the drug is licensed. Since securing approval for a drug can be a slow process, in practice the commercial patent life will be considerably less than twenty years (perhaps ten years) and the period is not necessarily free from competition, since other companies may seek to produce similar 'me-too' products that are nonetheless sufficiently different to secure their own patents. The latter is common within the industry. For instance, four of the current top ten companies currently produce their own cholesterol-lowering statin, with Pfizer's Lipitor the best-selling drug of all time. While the early statins like Lipitor are no longer in patent, companies are now introducing combination drugs with a statin as one component so as to secure new patents.

Along with patent protection, drugs are usually marketed under brand names that are simpler and easier to remember than chemical names and which help to secure a clear identity in the market and to improve sales, differentiating what may be chemically quite similar drugs. Lipitor is, for example, the brand name of atorvastatin. Brand names are protected by means of trademark registration that allows exclusive use of the name for a finite period, though this can quite readily be extended.

The most successful patented drugs change quite rapidly as new products come onto the market and existing drugs lose protection. The bestsellers by revenue in 2013 are shown in Table 10.3. Top of the list was Seretide, an inhaler, used in particular to treat asthma. Second was Humira, an anti-inflammatory medicine for conditions such as rheumatoid arthritis. This has generated such high sales value partly because of its expense (in the US, Humira costs around $1600 a month). Enbrel is another medicine that featured in the list in part because of its expense. Only one cholesterol-lowering statin, Crestor, remained in the 2013 top ten, although Lipitor, which now relies solely on its brand name, was still fourteenth in terms of sales value – its sales partly sustained by discounts and incentives for patients and insurers.

Bestsellers are typically drugs, particularly expensive drugs, for conditions held to require long-term medication. This may be because the conditions are often chronic, such as ulcers, asthma, diabetes, and depression. Alternatively, this may be because individuals, on the basis of some biomarker, are deemed to be at risk of possible subsequent illness. For instance, when high cholesterol is viewed as indicating individuals are at risk of a heart attack or a stroke, long-term medication is often recommended to try and

Table 10.3 Top ten pharmaceutical products, 2013

Product	Type of drug	Main treatment indication	Company	Sales 2012 (US$ billion)
Seretide/Advair	Corticosteroid + salmeterol	Asthma	GSK	8.9
Humira*	Monoclonal antibody	Auto-immune diseases	Abbott	8.5
Crestor	Statin	High cholesterol	AstraZeneca	8.3
Nexium	Proton pump inhibitor	Heartburn/stomach acid	AstraZeneca	7.5
Enbrel*	TNF inhibitor	Rheumatoid arthritis	Pfizer	7.5
Remicade*	Monoclonal antibody	Auto-immune diseases	Merck & Co.; Janssen Biotech	7.3
Abilify	Atypical antipsychotic	Schizophrenia; bipolar disorder	Bristol-Myers Squibb; Otsuka	7.0
Lantus*	Insulin analog	Diabetes	Sanofi	6.6
Mabthera*	Monoclonal antibody	Lymphomas and leukaemia	Genentech	6.0
Cymbalta	Serotonin-norepinephrine reuptake inhibitor	Major depressive disorder; general anxiety disorder	Eli Lilley	5.8

*Biopharmaceutical.

Source: IMS Health (2013).

reduce the risk. Such drugs have been termed 'drugs for life' (Dumit 2012), since once started, doctors often advise it is less risky to continue taking them than to stop, though patients may not continue to take them because they dislike the side-effects. Drugs that make over US$1 billion per annum in sales are termed 'blockbusters' and have been crucial to the industry. The search for blockbusters encourages large companies to focus on the health problems of more affluent countries (see commercial biases below) where sales are likely to be greater

Innovation, research and development, and biotechnology

Patent protection, which permits a higher price to be charged for a drug, is typically justified by the industry in terms of the high cost of the research and development (R&D) needed for product innovation. Leading companies spend between 15 and 16 per cent of revenue on R&D, although some spend rather more. Whether the R&D cost fully justifies the high prices for patented drugs remains a matter of debate. Certainly the cost of bringing drugs involving new molecular entities (NMEs) onto the market can be high, estimated at around $1300 million per drug for the top companies (Deloitte 2013), a figure that incorporates the development costs of drugs that do not secure approval. However, such figures are highly contested, not least because many new drugs are similar to those already on the market so the development costs may be lower. The US Food and Drug Administration (FDA) approves only a relatively small number of NMEs each year – between

20 and 30 per annum in the decade 2003–12 (Center for Drug Evaluation and Research 2103), with many applications for approval relating to generic medicines and some to biological products, including what are known as biosimilars, the 'me-toos' of the biological world. Moreover, pharmaceutical R&D may build on basic research, funded from the public purse, rather than by the companies themselves.

Increasingly, new drugs involve developments based on biological processes and some of the crucial R&D work is being done by smaller biotechnology companies, which, when a product with market potential is identified, may, if they lack the resources and expertise to secure regulatory approval and mount a successful market launch, then license it to a major pharmaceutical company. Alternatively, they may become takeover targets for multinational companies keen to secure new patented products. Such takeovers are common. For example, the highly successful California-based Genentech was taken over by the Swiss Hoffman La Roche in 2009. While many biotechnology companies are located in the USA and Europe, a growing number are found in countries such as Japan, Brazil, Argentina, and India.

The number of biotechnology products becoming bestsellers demonstrates the importance of the emerging biotechnology sector. The current top ten (see Table 10.3) includes five biopharmaceuticals: Humira, Enbrel, Remicade, Lantus, and Mabthera. In 2003, there was only one, Eprex, a drug to treat anaemia. Overall, the biotechnology market was worth almost US$282 billion in 2011.

Generic pharmaceuticals

Once a drug is out of patent, generic versions can be produced. The term generic can refer either to products or processes that are out of patent, or to those that do not have a trademark. Commonly the term refers to medicines produced once a patent ends, that are sold under their chemical rather than brand name, given that trademarks can be protected for longer than patents. For instance, once the patent for Prozac ended in 2001, generic versions began to be sold under the chemical name fluoxetine, since Eli Lilly retained the brand name as a registered trademark. While generating less revenue than patented drugs, generics represent a major source of sales volume. Given the cost of patented medicines, generics are essential to achieving global health aims, including universal health coverage and treatment for people living with HIV/AIDS.

The production of generic medicines has frequently been less attractive to leading companies than patented drugs since they are less profitable. Consequently, in the USA and Europe it has been largely left to specialist companies to produce them. However, some leading pharmaceutical companies are now putting much more emphasis on generics. For instance, Novartis has acquired several European generic companies in recent years and much of Teva's business is in generics. Furthermore, many of the companies in India and China concentrate on producing generics. The pharmaceutical industry in India is fragmented, with many small and medium enterprises and many of the manufacturing plants foreign-owned. Some leading companies successfully export generics to countries like the USA and Russia, seeking to secure approval from the FDA for the generic versions once patents are due to expire. The major companies include Sun Pharmaceuticals, the largest pharmaceutical company in India, which in 2014 moved to take over the mainly Japanese-owned Ranbaxy, and Dr Reddy's Laboratories, both of which produce generics for the US market. Interestingly, the FDA has started to inspect the manufacturing plants of foreign companies that produce pharmaceuticals for the US market, and in 2013 two Ranbaxy plants failed inspections, making them more vulnerable to takeover. China's industry has also been fragmented with around 3500 domestic pharmaceutical manufacturers, though this is a significant decline over the last decade. Domestic companies account for around 70 per cent of the Chinese market, with the top ten accounting for 20 per cent of that proportion. Some are engaged in joint ventures with foreign companies, in part as a way of circumventing China's strict import regulations. China, however, is currently a net exporter of pharmaceuticals, mostly to non-western countries, as well as a rapidly expanding market for medicines.

Activity 10.1

Look at the business section of a major national newspaper over a two-week period. Collect any stories about pharmaceutical companies. What can you observe about the companies or products covered?

Feedback

You may find that many of the companies are, or are affiliated with, the world's leading companies mentioned in this chapter. If trends in ownership, sales, profits or market growth are discussed, you may wish to think about such trends in relation to the global restructuring of the industry towards larger companies with worldwide reach.

How powerful is the pharmaceutical industry?

Light's (1995) framework that draws on the concept of countervailing powers is useful when assessing the power of the pharmaceutical industry. Countervailing powers are powers that stand in dynamic relation to one another so that if the power of one group or actor becomes dominant, it may elicit responses from others to try to redress this imbalance. Focusing on healthcare services, Light distinguishes four main actors: the medical profession, patients, the medico-industrial complex (commercial companies), and the state (government).

Figure 10.1 modifies and applies this model to the pharmaceutical industry, one type of commercial actor influencing health care. The figure directs us to consider the different relationships in which the industry is involved and to explore its power in each case. For instance, the medical profession is potentially an important countervailing power and could be a major independent force constraining the power of the industry. In general, however, the medical profession is largely supportive of the industry, since it relies heavily on the use of medicines for its own status and power; it is also subject to numerous blandishments from the industry. Similarly, governments have the potential to act as a countervailing power, regulating the industry through a range of mechanisms (see below). Governments can decide which drugs must be prescribed, which can be sold over the counter, and whether direct-to-consumer advertising is permitted. They can also attempt to control drug prices, and determine whether products should be approved and released onto the market. At the same time, as with the medical profession, they may be keen to support the industry, because of its contribution to the economy or to secure favourable access to products. Finally, patients can be a countervailing force, but their power tends to be limited unless operating collectively through users' groups.

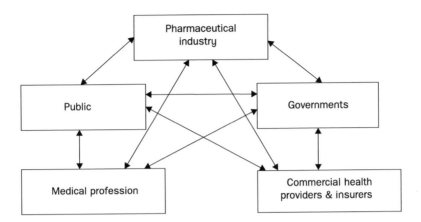

Figure 10.1 The pharmaceutical industry and countervailing powers

Source: Modified from Light (1995)

Mann's (1993) analysis of four sources of power is also useful for understanding the power of the pharmaceutical industry. He distinguishes between economic, political, ideological, and military power, but only the first three apply to the pharmaceutical industry. The industry's economic power is extensive, given the scale of the industry, the consolidation among leading companies, and its economic importance to the countries where companies are located. This was apparent when in 2004 the French Government made clear its preference for Sanofi-Synthelabo's bid for its sister French company, Aventis, over the possible bid from the Swiss company, Novartis. The industry's economic power can therefore also give it political power.

In addition, the industry has ideological power. This operates most obviously through the extensive marketing carried out by leading companies. This marketing activity is well documented. The USA and New Zealand are the only countries where direct-to-consumer advertising is officially permitted, and there is extensive and highly effective advertising through the mass media. Studies show that the most advertised brands are the most widely prescribed. In countries where such advertising is banned, product marketing is still extensive. Companies make considerable use of press releases about products and the illnesses they are intended to treat, often emphasizing how the illnesses can go undetected. Consequently, the public often learn about new products through newspapers, magazines, and television. Companies also encourage individuals to use simple online tests to identify whether they are at risk and should be taking some medicine. Moreover, direct marketing to doctors and other health professionals is pervasive. This includes advertisements in medical publications, sponsorship of meetings and research, provision of branded items, and personal contact by sales representatives. The amount leading companies spend on marketing is hotly debated, not least because the presentation of financial data in company reports makes this difficult to calculate. The industry typically suggests that the expenditure on marketing is lower than on R&D but more critical analysts have argued that it is far higher, with estimates as high as nearly a quarter of sales revenue (Gagnon and Lexchin 2008). Since regulatory controls are typically weaker in low-income countries, the potential ideological power of companies through publicity and marketing is particularly great despite the more limited purchasing power.

Activity 10.2

Obtain a copy of a major medical journal that accepts drug advertisements. Look at the drug products that are advertised in it and the language used to describe them. What proportion is for leading products? Who are the manufacturers? How do the advertisements encourage the use of different products?

Regulating the pharmaceutical industry

Regulating trade

The WTO is by far the most important organization regulating international trade, including trade in pharmaceuticals. As described in Chapters 3 and 8, it operates through periodically held trade negotiations and agreed multilateral agreements. One area of its work, particularly relevant to the industry, is intellectual property rights. The Agreement on Trade Related Aspects of Intellectual Property Rights (TRIPS), adopted in 1995, covers such matters as copyright, trademarks, geographical locations, and patents. It is designed to protect intellectual property rights across the world, although least-developed countries have until 2016 to put it fully into effect.

The agreement recognizes that patent protection can sometimes be overridden on public health grounds, for instance, when there are major epidemics. In these circumstances, a government may introduce 'compulsory licensing', permitting a local company to produce a patented product without the agreement of the patent owner. However, a country may do so only if they have first sought a voluntary licence from the patent holder, and must restrict use of the drug to the domestic market. The subsequent Doha Declaration, agreed in 2001, allows a country to issue a compulsory licence to import a drug from another country, if there is no domestic pharmaceutical industry, although some remuneration must be paid to the exporter. As discussed in the preceding chapter, since 2001 many countries have signed so-called 'TRIPS Plus' provisions as part of bilateral trade agreements, in particular with the USA. These limit their ability to use the flexibilities set out in the TRIPS agreement and often have stronger intellectual property protections than the original agreement. These changes to trade regulation are likely to have a significant impact on affordability and thus access to medication in low- and middle-income countries.

Regulating products and prices

Safety concerns about drug adulteration, side-effects, and the addictive properties of some medicines have led to the regulation of products that can be marketed and whether they require medical prescription. Drug approval agencies were only fully developed in western countries in the early 1960s, partly following the tragic consequences over the use of thalidomide, which heightened concerns about drug safety. An agency's task is to assess the benefits and risks of a drug as a treatment for a particular condition. Countries vary in the rigour of their approval agencies, and the extent to which they rely on prior judgements made by other agencies. Agencies review both patented and generic drugs before they can be released onto the market. They typically depend on the test results provided (and usually funded) by pharmaceutical companies, rather than their own research. The requirements for approving generic drugs are usually more limited than for drugs involving new molecular entities or new biological products.

Drug approval agencies mediate between the conflicting interests of pharmaceutical companies, which seek to make a profit and get products onto the market as quickly as possible, and the public who, while they may be interested in securing speedy access to a new treatment, have a strong interest in effectiveness and safety. Agencies have to deal with these conflicting interests on behalf of governments, which may also be torn between a desire to support the industry and the need to protect patients.

Agencies differ in their organizational structures, testing requirements, and assessment procedures. Among national agencies, the most important globally is the US FDA, given the importance of accessing the huge US market. The European Agency for the Evaluation of Medicinal Products (EMEA) now sets approval standards for EU countries. Its powers are presently limited, and approval is mandatory only for biotechnology and 'orphan' drugs (see below). Since the early 1990s, the International Conference on Harmonization (ICH) of Technical Requirements for the Registration of Pharmaceuticals for Human Use has been agreeing international guidelines on a range of matters concerning testing and clinical trials. There is some evidence that harmonization is leading to lower standards being set (Abraham and Reed 2001). The WHO is also beginning to play a part in commenting on the safety and effectiveness of drugs through the construction of essential drug lists largely for use in low-income countries.

Governments and healthcare organizations may also seek to regulate prices, since they often have to cover the costs of at least a proportion of medicines. In so doing, they may be anxious not to alienate the industry, especially if there are R&D or manufacturing facilities located within the country that contribute to the country's employment, wealth, and tax revenue. The precise mechanisms used to determine fair prices vary, and can sometimes be seen to favour the industry (Mossialos et al. 2004).

How effective is product regulation?

In considering the adequacy of regulatory arrangements for drug approval, two questions need to be addressed: Are the regulatory agencies independent of the pharmaceutical industry? And, are safety and effectiveness adequately assessed before a drug is released onto the market? On the question of independence, the key problem is that of *regulatory capture* (Abraham 1995), a process in which agencies take on the values and interests of the group whose activities it regulates. A number of factors facilitate such capture. One is the difficulty of finding the necessary expertise entirely independent of the industry to make assessments. Another is governments' desire to sustain and protect the industry. Moreover, some governments are politically sympathetic to large-scale businesses on ideological grounds.

On the question of the safety and effectiveness of drugs, the conclusion has to be that these are not fully assessed before a drug is released onto the market (Busfield 2006). This is recognized by the regulatory agencies themselves, in so far as they accept that further evaluation will be needed once the drug is licensed for the market and for various reasons do not want to delay its release. However, once approval is granted there is often little systematic testing of a drug using properly controlled trials unless this is required by the agency. The key limitations of testing are listed in Table 10.4. As a result, in many cases, problems with particular medicines only emerge after they have been on the market for some time. They may be withdrawn, or the advice on use changed significantly.

Table 10.4 The limitations of drug testing

Limitation	Problem
1. Lack of independent testing	Most testing is funded by the industry; when research is independent, results are usually less favourable to the tested drug (Kjaegard and Als-Nielson 2002)
2. Lack of transparency over test results	Unfavourable results may not be revealed by companies under the guise of commercial confidentiality
3. Companies decide how to handle trial withdrawals	Attrition affects trial results and can be used to make a drug look more effective
4. Limited number of human subjects tested	Tests usually involve a few thousand people and uncommon side-effects may not show up
5. Narrow range of human subjects	Most testing is on men and excludes women, children, and the elderly, yet a drug may be used for these groups even though they have different metabolisms
6. Narrow range of cases, with clearly defined illness	The boundaries of a drug's value are not tested, although the cost–benefit equation changes for more marginal cases
7. Companies select comparators and dosages to test	Can make a drug look more effective by using higher dosage of the tested drug or a low dosage of comparator
8. Companies select measures of effectiveness	Small differences that are not clinically significant can be presented as showing greater effectiveness
9. Testing mainly short term, usually no more than six months	Problems with long-term use will not show up
10. Blindness may be difficult to maintain	Visibility of some side-effects may mean researchers learn which subjects are on the active drug and which on the placebo
11. Limited systematic testing of interaction effects	Drugs are often taken alongside one another, especially among older people
12. Limited post-approval (Phase IV) testing	Need systematic research under conditions of normal clinical practice
13. Poor post-approval systems for reporting side-effects and adverse drug reactions	Adverse drug reactions and side-effects tend to be massively under-reported

For instance, the statin Baycol was voluntarily withdrawn in 2001, four years after it was first licensed in the USA, after it led to 31 deaths in the US alone (Furberg and Pitt 2001). The pain-reducing Vioxx, used in the treatment of arthritis, with sales of US$2.5 billion, was withdrawn in 2004 after its link to heightened risks of heart attacks was identified (McIntyre and Evans 2014). And the obesity drug Meridia was withdrawn in 2010 when a detailed study showed it increased the chances of a heart attack or stroke (Jorgensen et al. 2014). Full evaluation of a drug can take many years, with many people suffering side-effects and adverse drug reactions during this time.

A further issue is the use of individuals from low-income countries to test medicines that are then largely used in high-income countries. A classic example was the testing of the first contraceptive pill on Puerto Rican women. The practice exposes the trial subjects to the risks associated with a new product, which will have its major markets in more affluent countries. Moreover, drugs withdrawn from use in high-income countries may continue to be widely marketed in countries where drug approval is less stringent. Overall, the regulatory framework for the pharmaceutical industry remains variable at the national level, and somewhat nascent at the international level. If the industry continues to become globalized, this framework will need to be strengthened to better balance the interests of drug companies and users.

To what extent is the pharmaceutical industry becoming globalized?

In considering the extent to which the pharmaceutical industry is becoming globalized, it is helpful to distinguish the activities of trade, manufacturing, and product innovation. In terms of trade, the industry can be described as 'internationalized' given the many companies that sell products across the world. However, as Table 10.2 above indicates, the distribution of world sales revenue is uneven. Pharmaceutical trade is dominated by the leading companies selling to high-income countries. Western companies have also dominated trade in generic drugs, although there is growing trade among non-western countries and some of the largest of them are securing a foothold in western markets.

The liberalization of trade is somewhat uneven. Various developments have helped to open up trade, including moves to harmonize drug approval standards (see above) and the accession of more countries to the WTO. However, whether the enforcement of intellectual property rights facilitates or hinders trade remains subject to debate. Some argue that it constitutes a form of market imperfection on the supply side (Mossialos et al. 2004). Others contend it forms an important pillar of a global drug market.

Second, there is evidence of the internationalization of manufacturing. Although the headquarters of the ten leading companies are concentrated in a few countries, they manufacture their products in a range of countries. For example, AstraZeneca currently has 22 manufacturing sites in seventeen countries, including the UK, Sweden, France, Germany, Italy, the USA, Brazil, Puerto Rico, China, Japan, India, and Australia. GlaxoSmithKline largely manufactures at facilities in Europe and the USA, but also has plants in Puerto Rico, Singapore, and Australia.

Third, product innovation remains largely concentrated in western countries, although leading companies increasingly have some R&D operations in Asia. For instance, AstraZeneca's R&D is carried out in Sweden, the UK, and the USA, but also in Poland, Russia, Japan, India, and China. GlaxoSmithKline's R&D is carried out in the USA, the UK, Canada, Germany, France, Spain, and Belgium, but also in Singapore and China.

Overall, it is perhaps more accurate to say that there has so far largely been a process of westernization rather than globalization (Table 10.5). But the situation is changing towards globalization, as companies in China, Japan, and India become more important to global markets with their spending on pharmaceuticals increasing far more rapidly than in the USA and Europe (where there has been some stagnation following the financial crisis that began in 2007). Furthermore, the leading companies now often have at least one R&D facility in Asia. The industry does not yet transcend boundaries – globalization in its strictest sense – although the growing sale of drugs via the web may qualify as a form of transcendence.

Table 10.5 The pharmaceutical industry and globalization

Type of globalization	Extent
Internationalization – leading companies trade, manufacture, and innovate across the world	Pharmaceutical trade is extensive, but is largely asymmetrical flowing from the West; manufacturing is more international and product innovation is beginning to spread to non-western countries
Liberalization – reduction of trade barriers	Moves to harmonize drug approval standards, and accession to WTO reduces trade barriers, but patenting creates market imperfections
Globalization – transcendence of boundaries	While there are signs that production is delinked from geography, on the whole, consumption and product innovation are not

The consequences of a globalizing pharmaceutical industry

There are three main issues raised by an increasingly westernized pharmaceutical industry: the role of drugs in influencing health status; the need to correct commercial biases in the supply of drugs; and the inappropriate use of medicines.

Health status

In his classic study of the factors underpinning the long-term decline in mortality from infectious diseases in Britain from 1750 to 1950, McKeown (1976) argued that new vaccines and medicines made a relatively small contribution. The data for respiratory tuberculosis are given in Figure 10.2 and show that much of the decline occurred prior to the introduction of effective medical interventions. Rather, the first stage of the demographic transition, from high mortality and fertility to low mortality and fertility, predated the introduction of the relevant interventions. Instead, improvements in living standards were crucial. Subsequent writers have suggested that other factors, such as improvements in sanitation, were more important than general living standards. Yet they do not contradict McKeown's central point that medical interventions were less important than the broader social determinants of health.

Attention to the broad determinants of health does not mean, of course, that drug technologies do not contribute to the health of populations. One study contended that about half the increase in life expectancy in Britain since 1950 could be accounted for by medical care (Bunker 2001), but others have argued that this is an overestimate resulting from incorrect assumptions in the analysis. Furthermore, not all the benefits from drugs can be captured by changes in mortality. The reduction of pain and suffering is a major motivation for the use of medicines, as the continuing popularity of aspirin and paracetamol attests. Medicines can also shorten the duration of an illness, important for the quality of life of an individual as well as to society as a whole.

Commercial biases

As private businesses, pharmaceutical companies concentrate on producing drugs that are potentially profitable and this leads to biases in product portfolios. First, drugs used to treat chronic complaints are more attractive commercially than those for acute, more

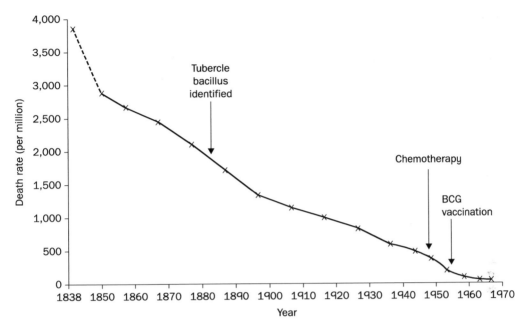

Figure 10.2 Respiratory tuberculosis death rates, England and Wales, 1838–1970

Source: McKeown (1976)

short-term illnesses, even if life-threatening. This is also the case with the increasing use of drugs to reduce the risks (often only minimally) of severe illnesses across large groups of people. Hence, as noted above, drugs for life dominate product development (see Table 10.3). Severe illnesses such as cancers are not entirely neglected and new medicines for treating cancer have come onto the market, but drugs for their treatment may not offer the same revenue potential because of the size of the groups involved unless very high prices are charged – something that is not entirely unusual. Second, rare illnesses tend to attract less attention, even if very serious, given the potentially small market for treatments. The extent of the problem of so-called 'neglected diseases' has led some countries to provide specific funding to the industry to develop 'orphan' drugs for rare conditions. In the USA, for example, measures were introduced in 1983 to make funding available to pharmaceutical companies for research on orphan drugs. It also introduced a procedure for getting a disease or condition formally approved as rare.

For low-income countries, the problem of commercial bias is even greater. Poorer countries have far fewer resources to spend on health care, including pharmaceuticals. Consequently, private companies have shown less interest in developing treatments for the health needs they face. For example, anti-malarial treatments are limited despite the disease killing around 660,000 people each year in the developing world. The cost of drugs is also a major hurdle for accessing appropriate medications in such countries. Although many of the drugs currently available are not patented, they remain beyond the resources of many low-income countries. This is not only a matter of the cost of drugs, but also of the absence of the necessary infrastructure to ensure their safe and effective use. Moreover, low-income countries are disadvantaged by the extension of intellectual property rights. On the one hand, the cost of new patented treatments is usually prohibitive, and countries are largely prevented from producing cheaper copies. On the other hand, indigenous natural substances used in a range of medicines, from which low-income countries might benefit, are being patented by pharmaceutical companies. It has been left to philanthropic entities, such as the Bill and Melinda Gates Foundation, to try and provide financial support for campaigns to eradicate certain major diseases, a form of philanthropic capitalism.

HIV/AIDS is an interesting case, since it has received more attention from leading pharmaceutical companies than other diseases common in low-income countries. This is undoubtedly because the disease also affects affluent countries. Many leading companies have drugs for HIV and AIDS, but existing treatments are oriented to strains prevalent in industrialized countries. Companies protect these drugs using patents, and have been slow to make them more readily available at reduced prices or by waiving patent protection. There has been relatively little private investment to develop a vaccine for HIV and AIDS.

From an ethical perspective, it is clearly unacceptable to leave the health needs of the developing world to the profit-seeking motives of the commercial market. Moreover, neglect of these needs is likely to prove short-sighted in an increasingly globalized world. The combined use of incentives and regulation by governments and international organizations is clearly needed to address these commercial biases.

The inappropriate use of medicines

A third consequence of a globalizing pharmaceutical industry is the emergence of forces that encourage the inappropriate use of medicines. Amid increasing pressures to market drugs worldwide, drugs may be prescribed unnecessarily in a range of circumstances. One is where an individual's condition is not especially severe and the possible side-effects outweigh the benefits. Another is where a drug is prescribed, even when there is evidence that the condition is not responsive to that drug. The misuse of antibiotics to treat viral infections is an example and is not restricted to western countries. China has, for instance, high levels of antibiotic use, widely recognized in the health field as excessive, in part occasioned by various structural incentives for prescribing. Such patterns of misuse have global consequences in the form of growing drug resistance. Another is where a drug is prescribed in a high dosage when a lower dosage would be almost as effective and have fewer side-effects. Yet another is when a drug that is initially necessary then continues to be prescribed even though it is no longer needed, increasing the chances of side-effects. The globalization of the pharmaceutical market ahead of appropriate prescribing protocols and guidelines across all countries, or with guidelines that set thresholds for use far too low, or where there are clear incentives for prescribing, gives rise to individual and collective risks.

🖉 Activity 10.3

The fifth edition of the American Psychiatric Association's *Diagnostic and Statistical Manual of Mental Disorders* (2013) has added a binge eating disorder. Is this an instance of medicalization? Is it desirable for individuals to try to reduce their weight by taking medications?

Feedback

You may have considered that defining binge eating as a mental disorder creates a need and legitimacy for medication. Medication or an emphasis on medicines may also de-prioritize an emphasis on the environment and social determinants that have been shown to be so important in creating ill health.

Summary

The pharmaceutical industry has undergone significant change in recent decades. In particular, the market for pharmaceuticals, while still dominated by western countries, is witnessing by far the largest expansion in China, India, and Latin America – expansion that reflects more rapid economic growth in these countries and the lower levels of pharmaceutical use in the past. Leading western companies still have a large share of the market, but despite continuing mergers and acquisitions to increase their size, this is no greater than twenty years ago. However, overall the industry has considerable power and regulation of the industry by governments is not especially tight. Pharmaceutical companies are especially skilful at marketing their products both to doctors and the public and in encouraging the demand for and use of medicines, sometimes beyond appropriate levels. Their commercial character is reflected in their continuing emphasis on products for common chronic conditions or those designed to reduce the risk of subsequent illness, products that are likely to be the most profitable, and in their relative neglect of the life-threatening diseases of low-income countries.

This chapter has also discussed the extent to which the pharmaceutical industry is shaped by trade regulations that lie outside of the national remit and that promote and protect the current model of research and manufacturing. It highlights the extent to which the market for global pharmaceuticals and access to medicines are governed by global factors. Efforts to address challenges in regulation, access, development or marketing of medication need to consider these systemic issues.

References

Abraham, J. (1995) *Science, Politics and the Pharmaceutical Industry: Controversy and Bias in Drug Regulation*. London: UCL Press.

Abraham, J. and Reed, T. (2001) Trading risks for markets: the international harmonisation of pharmaceuticals regulation, *Health Risk and Society*, 3: 113–28.

American Psychiatric Association (2013) *Diagnostic and Statistical Manual of Mental Disorders* (5th edn.). Washington, DC: American Psychiatric Association.

Bunker, J.P. (2001) The role of medical care in contributing to health improvements within societies, *International Journal of Epidemiology*, 30: 1260–3.

Busfield, J. (2003) Globalization and the pharmaceutical industry revisited, *International Journal of Health Services*, 33: 581–605.

Busfield, J. (2006) Pills, power, people: sociological understanding of the pharmaceutical industry, *Sociology*, 40: 297–314.

Center for Drug Evaluation and Research (2013) *Novel New Drugs Summary, 2012*. Washington, DC: Center for Drug Evaluation and Research.

Deloitte UK Centre for Health Solutions (2013) *Measuring the Return from Pharmaceutical Innovation*. London: Deloitte.

Dumit, J. (2012) *Drugs for Life: How Pharmaceutical Companies Define Our Health*. Durham, NC: Duke University Press.

Furberg, C. and Pitt, B. (2001) Withdrawal of cerivastatin from the world market, *Current Controlled Trial in Cardiovascular Medicine*, 2 (5): 205–7.

Gagnon, M.-A. and Lexchin, J. (2008) The cost of pushing pills: a new estimate of pharmaceutical promotion expenditures in the United States, *PLoS Medicine*, 5 (1): e1.

IMS Health (2013) *Global Rankings 2012*. Collegeville, PA: IMS Health.

Jorgensen, M.E., Torp-Pedersen, C., Finer, N., Caterson, I., James, W.P., Legler, U.F. et al. (2014) Association between serum bilirubin and cardiovascular disease in an overweight high risk population from the SCOUT trial, *Nutrition, Metabolism and Cardiovascular Disease*, 24 (6): 656–62.

Kjaegard, L.L and Als-Nielson, B. (2002) Association between competing interests and authors' conclusions: epidemiological study of randomised clinical trials published in the BMJ, *British Medical Journal*, 325: 249–52.

Light, D. (1995) Countervailing powers: a framework for professions in transition, in T. Johnson, G. Larkin and M. Saks (eds) *Health Professions and the State in Europe*. London: Routledge.

Mann, M. (1993) *The Sources of Social Power*, Vol. II: *The Rise of Classes and Nation States, 1760–1914*. Cambridge: Cambridge University Press.

McIntyre, W.F. and Evans, G. (2014) The Vioxx[R] legacy: enduring lessons from the not so distant past, *Cardiology Journal*, 21 (2): 203–5.

McKeown, T. (1976) *The Modern Rise of Population*. London: Edward Arnold.

Mossialos, E., Mrazek, M. and Walley, T. (eds) (2004) *Regulating Pharmaceuticals in Europe: Striving for Efficiency, Equity and Quality*. Milton Keynes: Open University Press.

Tarabusi, C. and Vickery, G. (1998) Globalization in the pharmaceutical industry: Parts I and II, *International Journal of Health Services*, 28: 67–105, 282–303.

Globalization and non-communicable diseases

11

Helen Walls and Neil Pearce

Overview

In this chapter, you will learn about the challenge of non-communicable disease globally, and the impact of globalization on our lifestyles and on the associated risk factors for non-communicable disease.

Learning objectives

After working through this chapter, you will be able to:

- describe how globalization affects the global burden of non-communicable disease
- describe how globalization affects the global burden of risk factors for non-communicable disease
- understand how globalization, including trade liberalization, is driving the underlying changes affecting non-communicable diseases

Key terms

Agricultural subsidies: Payments by governments to agricultural producers for the purpose of stabilizing food prices, managing the supply of agricultural commodities, supporting farmers' incomes, and strengthening the agricultural sector.

Multinational corporation (MNC): A corporation that is registered in more than one country or that has operations in more than one country, both producing and selling goods or services in those countries.

Trade liberalization: The process whereby a country opens up its markets to international trade by reducing taxes (known as tariffs) and other limits (such as quotas) on goods coming in and out. It also increasingly includes rights for investors, pressures to privatize as well as imposed regulatory changes to comply with international standards.

Transnational corporation (TNC): A corporation that differs from a multinational corporation, in that it does not identify with one national home. While traditional MNCs are national companies with foreign subsidiaries, TNCs spread out their operations in many countries, which improves local responsiveness.

Introduction

Non-communicable disease (NCD) (also known as 'chronic disease') has emerged in recent decades as the leading cause of death, and disease burden, in high- and in low- and middle-income countries alike. Longer life expectancy and therefore an ageing population are main factors in this, but aspects of globalization are also having a marked impact on this increase.

While there is no universally accepted definition for NCDs, they are generally diseases of relatively long duration and slow progression that are non-infectious, but they may be caused by infectious agents (e.g. hepatitis B and C infection is a cause of liver cancer). The main types, based on their contributions to mortality, are heart disease, stroke, cancer, diabetes, and chronic respiratory disease. However, when morbidity is also taken into account, other conditions such as neurological disease, mental health disorders, musculoskeletal disorders, and hearing loss are also of major importance. Once considered 'diseases of affluence', the burden of NCD in developing countries is now considered substantial. Globally, more than 60 per cent of deaths and almost 50 per cent of the healthy life 'lost' to illness (as measured in disability-adjusted life years, DALYs) are reportedly due to NCDs. In 2008, about 80 per cent of NCD deaths reportedly occurred in low- and middle-income counties, up from 40 per cent in 1990. Figure 11.1 illustrates this burden of NCD across country income levels.

Some authors, however (notably Katz 2013), suggest that such figures (which become notably less striking when population size is taken into account, for example) misrepresent the actual burden of NCD. These authors suggest the actual burden of NCD in low- and middle-income countries is considerably smaller, and that the misleading nature of the often-reported statistics favours globalized corporate interests.

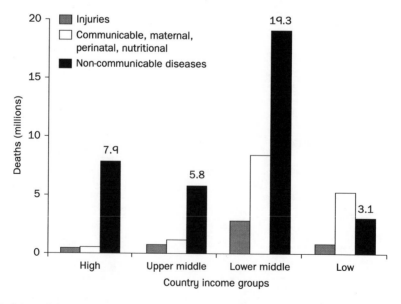

Figure 11.1 Cause of death across countries, by World Bank income group, 2008

Source: Beaglehole et al. (2011)

Risk factors for NCDs include tobacco use, harmful use of alcohol, physical inactivity, unhealthy diets, occupational and environmental exposures, and infection. Many of these are considered preventable, but their underlying causes are complex and becoming increasingly globalized. For example, with NCDs relating to poor diets and nutrition, an underlying cause is the powerful food/beverage and tobacco multinational and trans-national corporations, and the challenge of regulating their products as discussed in detail in Chapters 8 and 9.

Between modifiable NCD risk factors and NCDs, there are 'intermediate risk factors', which include overweight/obesity and elevated blood glucose, blood pressure, and cho-lesterol. Secondary prevention measures to address these include changes in diet or physical activity, the use of medicines to control blood pressure, cholesterol, and blood sugar levels, and pharmacological/surgical means to address obesity. Intervening on established intermediate risk factors is important, but it is particularly desirable (and potentially cost-effective) to reduce vulnerability to developing such disease.

Non-communicable diseases have major adverse social, economic, and health effects. Half of those who die of NCDs are in their prime productive years, with a quarter of all NCD deaths occurring below the age of 60. Every 10 per cent rise in NCD prevalence is associated with a 0.5 per cent reduction in rates of annual economic growth (Stuckler 2008). The accumulated impact of this is substantial.

To date, the resources applied to meet the NCD challenge at global level have been small, particularly compared with the considerable resources given by some countries to combat NCDs at national level. For example, the World Health Organization (WHO) budget for NCDs in 2006 was less than 5 per cent. However, the political priority accorded NCDs is increasing.

In September 2011, a United Nations High Level Meeting on the Prevention and Control of Non-Communicable Disease (UN HLM on NCDs) was held. This is only the second time a UN HLM has been dedicated to a health topic (the first being on HIV/AIDS in 2001). At the meeting, UN member states committed to a comprehensive set of actions to prevent and treat NCDs, with a specific goal to strengthen national multi-sectoral plans by the end of 2013. The need to address social determinants of NCDs was reiterated at the 64th World Health Assembly held in Geneva, Switzerland, in May 2011 by WHO member states in preparation for the UN HLM in 2011. In July 2013, European Ministers of Health renewed their commitment to address the NCD burden at the WHO Ministerial Conference on Nutrition and Non-communicable Diseases in the Context of Health 2020 by adopting a new declaration – the Vienna Declaration on Nutrition and Non-communicable Diseases in the Context of Health 2020. The Vienna Declaration has a focus on improving nutrition and physical activity levels, and argues that influential policies initiated in sectors outside of health will be important in addressing premature death from NCD.

Impact of globalization on traditional risk factors

The key modifiable risk factors that increase the risk of most NCDs, according to the current WHO website on NCDs, are tobacco use, physical inactivity, unhealthy diet, and the harmful use of alcohol. The direct health effects of globalization on NCD prevalence, via these factors, are illustrated by the increasingly globalized production, marketing, and consumption (facilitated by trade liberalization and increases in foreign direct investment as discussed in Chapter 9) of tobacco, alcohol, processed food products, and energy-saving technologies, particularly influential here being the motor car. These commodities now reach most parts of most countries. Advertisers use increasingly sophisticated

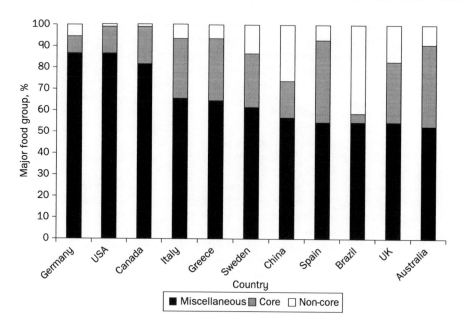

Figure 11.2 Proportion of major food groups advertised to children, by country, 2007–08

Source: Kelly et al. (2010)

means to influence our desire for and consumption of such products, often taking advantage of weak regulatory environments. A significant proportion of global marketing targets children. Figure 11.2 illustrates the nature of food advertising to children, in that in all countries shown, 'non-core' (read: unhealthy, processed) foods make up the majority of foods advertised.

Tobacco use

Tobacco use is an important risk factor common to major NCDs, including coronary heart disease, stroke, chronic obstructive pulmonary disease, and lung cancer. It causes one in six of all NCD deaths, and accounts for 30 per cent of cancers globally. Almost 6 million people die from tobacco use each year, both through direct use and second-hand smoke. In low- and middle-income countries, increasingly high rates of tobacco use are projected to lead to a doubling of the number of tobacco-related deaths between 2010 and 2030.

Transnational tobacco companies aggressively exploit the potential for growth in tobacco sales, deliberately subverting tobacco control efforts, including those of the WHO. Tobacco control in developed countries – in the form of increased tobacco taxes, restrictions on advertising of tobacco, and bans on smoking in public places – has resulted in marked reductions in tobacco sales and consumption. But the industry is now exploiting the opportunities offered by the development of electronic cigarettes to circumvent advertising restrictions and re-normalize the appearance of smoking. Simultaneously, the tobacco industry is shifting its promotional activities to low- and middle-income countries, exploiting their weaker regulatory environments to use marketing strategies that have been banned in many developed countries (see also the discussions in Chapter 9).

Physical inactivity

Approximately 30 per cent of the world's population does not meet minimum recommendations for physical activity. Despite some positive trends in leisure-time (discretionary) physical activity – which in fact accounts for only a small part of total physical energy expenditure – the prevalence of incidental, transportation-related, and occupational physical activity is falling. Between 6 and 10 per cent of mortality from NCD worldwide can be attributed to physical inactivity, and this percentage is even higher for specific diseases (e.g. 30 per cent for ischaemic heart disease). In 2007, about 5 million deaths globally from NCD could have been prevented if inactive people had instead been sufficiently active. Physical inactivity is a risk factor for NCD independent of its effect on body size/ shape.

In recent decades, energy expenditure has decreased markedly, and lifestyles have become more sedentary. Leisure-time physical activity (e.g. sport, running, going to the gym) only accounts for a small part of total physical energy expenditure, and it would be unlikely to offset these reductions in physical activity. Energy expenditure has declined due to greater use of energy-saving devices, and most importantly, changes to the urban environment, including urban design, safety concerns (which discourage children from walking to school, for example), the rise of the car (which causes further concern about the safety of children walking), and the near demise of public transport (a particular concern in low- and middle-income countries).

Unhealthy diets

Nutrition is an important risk factor for NCD, with diets high in fats, salt and sugar and low in fruits, vegetables and whole grains particularly problematic. Such diets, which are becoming increasingly common, are associated with overweight, obesity, and NCDs such as heart disease, diabetes, and some cancers. Poor diet quality is also associated with micronutrient deficiency, such as vitamin A deficiency, a leading cause of childhood blindness in low-income countries. As a result of these developments, overweight and obesity, and associated health problems, already well established in high-income countries, are also on the rise in low- and middle-income countries, affecting more than two-thirds of adults in many countries. In the Pacific, the prevalence of obesity is among the world's highest, and type 2 diabetes affects up to 30 per cent of adults (before the Second World War it was virtually unknown). Approximately 18 per cent of deaths worldwide are attributable to raised blood pressure, which is largely due to dietary salt intake.

With diets and nutrition, these processes are driving a 'nutrition transition' from traditional diets rich in fruit, vegetables, and grains towards increasingly processed diets, and diets with a high proportion of saturated fat, salt, and sugars. Such foods have become cheap, readily available, and enticing to consumers. A fast food culture has taken hold in many countries. The terms 'Coca-colonization' and 'McDonaldization' have been coined to describe the impact of the western, and predominantly American, culture on developing countries.

Harmful use of alcohol

Excessive alcohol use has been linked to NCDs, including many cancers (of the oral cavity, pharynx, larynx, oesophagus, liver and female breast, for example), liver cirrhosis, and cardiovascular disease.

Alcohol can be made from a wide variety of agricultural inputs, and is produced both formally and informally throughout the world. But the transnational alcohol industry is growing in power. As with many other globalized industries, a few large companies dominate the market. The ten largest alcoholic beverage marketers accounted for 48 per cent of sales (by volume) of globalized brands in 2005 (see also the discussion in Chapter 9 for more detail on alcohol industry ownership).

The traditional risk factors considered key to NCD mortality have also been recently conceptualized in the proposed five-target '25x25' strategy – which aims to reduce mortality from NCDs by 25 per cent by 2025 – now incorporated into the WHO's Global NCD Action Plan 2013–2020. The strategy was partly derived from the UN HLM on NCDs, and has been publicized as the most effective strategy to tackle NCDs globally. The ultimate goal is to decrease mortality from four diseases (cardiovascular disease, diabetes, cancer, and chronic respiratory disease) by 25 per cent by the year 2025. Its five targets (four risk factors and one cardiovascular preventive drug treatment) are:

• accelerate tobacco control*
• reduce dietary salt consumption*
• treat people at high risk of cardiovascular disease*
• reduce alcohol consumption
• reduce physical inactivity

(*These are considered the highest-priority interventions, which if applied rigorously, will achieve the 25x25 goal.)

The limitations to this traditional approach, including the 25x25 strategy, will be discussed in the next section.

✏️ **Activity 11.1**

1 Consider a food item you ate for dinner last night, and its likely country of origin. Now, on a piece of paper, try to list as many stages as possible the food item might have gone through, from production to eventual consumption by you.
2 How do you think your food supply chain might be changing as a consequence of globalization? Have there been changes in recent years to the foods that you are able or not able to buy? Have there been changes in availability, quality, packaging, variety, sources or cost of certain foodstuffs?

Feedback

1 Your answer might look something like Figure 11.3.

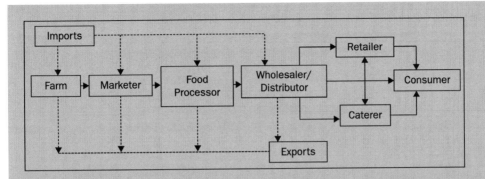

Figure 11.3 Food supply chains

Source: Dani and Deep (2010)

2 You may have noted some of the following changes:

Increase in availability of ready-made meals and convenience foods	Less home cooking
Increase in availability of organic foods, and its reduction in price	Changes in variety, diversity, and availability
More local food but fewer local shops	Changes to prevalence of food poverty
Changes in food technologies/food markets	Easier choice (labels and information)
More specialized food markets	Changes in food prices
More supermarkets	Increases in branding

Limitations of the traditional approach

A key limitation of the '25x25' strategy outlined above is that it seeks to reduce preventable mortality, but ignores the large burden of morbidity from NCDs. The NCDs addressed by the 25x25 strategy (cardiovascular disease, diabetes, cancer, and chronic respiratory disease) account for a very high proportion of total NCD deaths (87 per cent in the most recent Global Burden of Disease report), but for only fifty-four per cent of NCD when morbidity and disability are also taken into account.

When the burden of disease is measured as disability-adjusted life years (DALYs), incorporating information on both mortality and morbidity, a different picture emerges. In addition to the four diseases addressed by this strategy, other conditions that have high prevalence and involve a large burden of disability, but are not included in the 25x25 strategy, include mental disorders such as depressive disorders and schizophrenia, neurological disease and musculoskeletal disease, as well as visual impairment and hearing loss. Musculoskeletal diseases, for example, can severely reduce a person's ability to undertake manual labour, such as farming – the dominant productive activity in rural settings that are home to 50 per cent of the world's population.

A focus on morbidity not only changes the list of 'key diseases', it also changes the list of 'key exposures', since most cases of mental disorders, neurological disease, and musculoskeletal disease are not caused by the risk factors targeted by the 25×25 strategy. Other 'missing causes' include infections, occupational exposures, and environmental exposures. However, these exposures to individual lifestyle, occupational and environmental risk factors are shaped by the structural (distal) or more 'upstream' determinants (i.e. the 'causes of the causes'), which create the context in which the more proximal risk factors emerge. Some key examples of such determinants include urban design, poverty and inequality, unemployment, air pollution, and climate change. The narrow focus of the 'traditional approach' to addressing NCDs only deals with about half the NCD burden, and would prevent about a third of the problem.

✎   **Activity 11.2**

Why do you think the 'traditional approach' for addressing risk factors for NCDs may have become popular? Make a few notes based on what you have read so far. Draw on your own experience too, if you think it relevant.

Feedback

Some of the reasons you thought of might include:

* Failure to consider alternative approaches to measuring the NCD burden and address risk factors.
* Ease of addressing limited number of risk factors and diseases.
* There are clear individual-level (behavioural) risk factors associated with the traditional approach, which are easier to address than more 'upstream' determinants or the 'causes of the causes'.
* Easier to galvanize support around a narrower agenda.

Impact of globalization on NCD risk factors

In addition to their impacts on the 'traditional' NCD risk factors, many aspects of globalization are also having a substantial impact on the 'missing causes' of NCD, and the structural or underlying causes. Some of these impacts are discussed below.

Infections

Infection in early life increases the risk of NCDs in later life, and in adult life combinations of NCDs and infections, such as diabetes and tuberculosis, can interact adversely. An estimated one in six cancers globally are caused by treatable or preventable infections – the four main infections (human papilloma virus, *Helicobacter pylori*, hepatitis B and C viruses) accounting for two million annual cases of cervical, gut, and liver cancers globally. In addition to increasing transmission risk through increasing flows of people between regions, today's global trading system, with the traded large volumes of diverse products, amplified the transmission of infections. In the case of novel infections with long incubation periods, such as the human immunodeficiency virus (HIV) or variant Creutzfeld Jacob Disease (vCJD), this transmission can disseminate the infection to distant populations well in advance of detection.

Occupational and environmental exposures

Liberalization of trade has had benefits for workers, such as through the spread of human rights in employment law, but such liberalization has also been accompanied by a transfer of obsolete and hazardous technologies, chemicals, processes and waste, including asbestos and pesticides no longer produced or used in industrialized countries, jeopardizing the health of workers. Globalization has also been accompanied by an increased frequency of occupational accidents in developing countries. The movement of capital and technology, and changes in work organization appear to have outpaced the systems for protecting workers' health.

However, the causes discussed are shaped by the structural (distal) or more upstream determinants. The effects of globalization on economic and financial factors, trade policy, and climate change are discussed below.

Economic and financial factors

The indirect effects of globalization are mediated by economic and financial factors such as changes in household income, government expenditure, the availability and price of commodities, and the rules that regulate these. Such changes are often themselves driven by trade liberalization in the form of more liberal trade agreements between countries, and they influence household access to commodities associated with NCD risk or protective effects. National income influences public sector resources available for public health and health services.

Trade protectionism and liberalization

Agricultural policies that give preference to domestic producers through protective measures are likely to influence NCD prevalence. For example, the likely domestic effects of the US and European Union (EU) agricultural subsidies are reduced consumption and favourable NCD outcomes through sustaining higher prices, while at the same time they limit competition from primary producers of fresh produce in developing countries, reducing the ability of these countries to improve their national incomes through trade. The trade liberalization associated with globalization leads, at least in theory, to substantial benefits such as economic growth, but there is evidence to suggest it also results in poorer health outcomes in countries over a certain income level, and that it exacerbates inequities between and within countries – inequity and poverty are both 'upstream' risk factors for NCD.

Climate change

Climate change, the classic example of a globalized environmental problem, is also likely to increase NCD risk. With climate change, extreme weather events such as severe heat waves, droughts, storms, and floods will become more frequent and more severe. This will increase many risks to human health, and exacerbate the incidence of some NCDs, including cardiovascular disease, some cancers, respiratory health, mental disorders, injuries, and malnutrition.

Intervention approaches

There are a number of ways to address the NCD risk at a variety of levels. An approach that many advocate, particularly with regard to dietary choices, tobacco and alcohol use, emphasizes the role of individual choice and responsibility, and interventions aimed at educating people to make healthier choices. However, there is little evidence that such proximal or 'downstream' interventions really work. Furthermore, they must be undertaken and paid for by each generation, which is expensive and time-consuming. They also tend to exacerbate health inequalities more than 'upstream' population interventions because they are preferentially adopted by those with the resources that will help make healthy choices. They are also of little relevance to addressing some of the determinants of NCD risk over which even advocates of this approach would concede affected individuals have little control – NCD risks from air pollution, for example. While for some population subgroups (particularly those with established disease) individual-level lifestyle interventions may sometimes be beneficial, at a population level such interventions are not enough.

Underlying the NCD risk factors, including those 'non-traditional' risk factors such as infections, occupational and environmental exposures, are the more distal or 'upstream' determinants of NCDs and their behavioural risk factors. These include urban design, poverty and inequality, unemployment, social instability, trade agreements, air pollution, and climate change. Interventions to address these are potentially more effective, longer-lasting and more equitable. An example of such a measure that has worked is a substantial fall in blood cholesterol levels in Mauritius, not brought about by health education or drugs, but by negotiating trade agreements that enabled imported cooking oil to switch from largely palm oil (high in saturated fatty acids) to almost wholly lean oil. However, few such interventions have been enacted, perhaps because they often lie outside the health sector.

In most countries, government agencies outside health have resisted attempts from ministries and departments of health to influence their policies. Furthermore, global rules and power imbalances constrain the ability of countries and national health services to respond adequately to health problems. Politicians are generally reluctant to support structural changes that might threaten certain powerful industries, the food and car industries, for example. Where they have attempted to influence industry, it has largely been on a voluntary basis, or what is termed 'self-regulation'. But evidence suggests that these voluntary agreements are selective, difficult to evaluate, and often breached. With the shaping of international trade rules the influence of national governments has been limited by insufficient resources, expertise, and technical support. Furthermore, whereas trade liberalization through trade agreements used to be about removing barriers to trade, it is increasingly addressing non-tariff barriers, areas not formerly part of the trade regime. These changes are enabling greater industry involvement in policy-making, and eroding domestic policy space and national sovereignty, as we have seen in the discussions in Chapters 4 and 5, which focus on global health and its governance and the role of actors, including states within this.

Effective intervention addressing NCDs is challenging, and requires careful planning, political support, and appropriate infrastructure. Advocates, too, should be cognisant that many of the upstream solutions that address NCDs are also positive from other perspectives, such as for the environment or climate change. It may also be useful to work with advocates of these causes to generate and tackle common-cause agendas. As we have seen in other chapters in this book, and in other volumes in the UPH series, health is just a part of the policy mix, and people often will not vote for individual healthy lifestyle interventions, or to have their lifestyle options restricted solely for some potential future health benefit. However, they will vote for safe liveable neighbourhoods and cities, in which it is easy to walk or cycle to work or school, and in which locally produced food is widely available and affordable. In short, people may support healthy environmental changes for non-health reasons.

 Activity 11.3

Marketing activities can be classified into '5Ps':

- Product: creating and diversifying products.
- Price: the price of the product and how it will affect customers.
- Place: the availability of the product (distribution) and location of sales points.
- Promotion: activities such as market entry marketing, advertising, sales promotions, websites.
- People: promoting the brand to those who might buy it; associating it with TV programmes, movies, sports, music and events, competitions and philanthropy.

In your country, list the ways in which fast food, soft drink, alcohol or cigarette companies are using the 5Ps to promote their product. Do you think these strategies are succeeding in changing the choices of those around you?

Feedback

You may have noticed that there are now many more different brands offering essentially the same product, but in many different versions. For example, light or differently flavoured versions of soft drinks or chocolate bars sold in different formats. You may also have noticed the extent to which celebrities or sports events are used to promote food, alcohol, and cigarettes to create an association between these and the products sold.

Summary

You have seen how globalization is having a complex impact on the risk factors for NCDs. One aspect is unequivocal: the increasing influence of massive multinational and transnational corporations on NCD risk factors, through the globalization and marketing of particular products. The problems with addressing NCD at an individual-level, and the 'upstream' nature of many determinants of NCD suggest that effective interventions for NCD will take place at policy level, often nationally or internationally, and will include sectors outside of what is traditionally considered health.

References

Beaglehole, R., Bonita, R., Alleyne, G., Horton, R., Li, L., Lincoln, P. et al. (2011) UN High-Level Meeting on Non-Communicable Diseases: addressing four questions, *The Lancet*, 378 (9789): 449–55.

Dani, S. and Deep, A. (2010) Fragile food supply chains: reacting to risks, *International Journal of Logistics Research and Applications*, 13 (5): 395–410.

Katz, A.R. (2013) Noncommunicable diseases: global health priority or market opportunity? An illustration of the World Health Organization at its worst and at its best, *International Journal of Health Services*, 43 (3): 437–58.

Kelly, B., Halford, J.C.G., Boyland, E.J., Chapman, K., Bautista-Castano, I., Berg, C. et al. (2010) Television food advertising to children: a global perspective, *American Journal of Public Health*, 100 (9): 1730–6.

Stuckler, D. (2008) Population causes and consequences of leading chronic diseases: a comparative analysis of prevailing explanations, *Milbank Quarterly*, 86: 273–326.

Globalization and infectious diseases   12

Marco Liverani

Overview

In this chapter, we explore the links between globalization and infectious diseases. In the first section, we highlight areas in which evidence suggest that globalizing processes have had an impact on the emergence or spread of infections. We then look at the historical development of global mechanisms for infectious disease prevention and control up to the present, identifying key elements of change and continuity.

Learning objectives

After working through this chapter, you will be able to:

- understand ways in which globalizing processes have affected infectious disease risk and dynamics
- recognize changing patterns and approaches in global mechanisms for infectious disease prevention and control
- consider challenges and opportunities in the past and present context of global policy and initiatives

Key terms

Emerging infectious diseases: Diseases that have appeared in a population for the first time, or that may have existed previously but are rapidly increasing in incidence or geographic range.

GOARN (Global Outbreak Alert and Response Network): An international collaboration of technical partners worldwide in the area of epidemic alert and response, based at the WHO in Geneva, including public sectors, inter-governmental organizations, non-governmental organizations, and the private sector.

International Health Regulations: An international instrument that is legally binding on all WHO member states, and aims to protect against the international spread of disease, avoiding unnecessary interference with international traffic and trade.

The impact of globalization on infectious disease risk

Globalization is a complex set of social, economic, technological, political, and cultural developments that have created new connections and interdependencies between people, places, and environments. Some of those developments may have important effects on infectious disease risk and dynamics, given their potential to influence in various ways whether a pathogen can survive, evolve, infect susceptible hosts, and cause disease

(Saker et al. 2007). The link between globalization and infectious diseases can be observed most directly in changing patterns of human mobility. Population movements have been a source of disease transmission throughout human history, as microbes have always travelled with human carriers and other vectors along trade, migratory, and military routes. Over the past two centuries, the globalizing force of commerce and advances in transport technologies have contributed to a dramatic expansion and growth of international travel, creating new opportunities for the rapid spread of communicable diseases across wide geographic areas. During the nineteenth century, for example, cholera spread widely along the increasingly interconnected trade routes, from India to China and from Europe to the United States, becoming the first truly global disease. In 1832, a British journalist noted that cholera 'mastered every variety of climate, surmounted every natural obstacle, conquered every people' (in Briggs 1961: 76). From the post-war period to the present, progress in public health and medicine has reduced the rates of illness and mortality from infectious diseases, especially in high-income countries; yet, new public health challenges have resulted from the unprecedented increase in human mobility, driven by several factors, including the development of air, sea, and land transport, the growth of tourism and business travel, conflicts and civil unrests, structural changes in the global economy, and greater liberalization of markets and migration policies. Notably, the increasingly high volume of international air traffic has greatly enhanced the risk of communicable disease transmission across countries. In 1960, there were about 70 million international journeys globally, but by 2004 the number exceeded 760 million (Gushulak and MacPherson 2006). At present, about 3 billion air passengers are carried in one year, and estimates indicate that in 2030 the number might reach 6.4 billion (ICAO 2014). The rapid spread of severe acute respiratory syndrome (SARS) in 2003 exemplifies the public health implications of these trends. SARS is a respiratory infection caused by a novel coronavirus, which is believed to have crossed the species barrier recently from animals to humans. The first case of SARS was identified in Guangdong Province, China, in November 2002. The disease was carried out of Guangdong Province in February 2003, when an infected physician spent a night in a hotel in the Hong Kong district of Kowloon, one of the most densely populated areas in the world. By the end of February, the disease began spreading globally along air travel routes as guests at the same hotel flew home to Canada, Singapore, and other countries (Ruan et al. 2006). As of August 2003, when the World Health Organization (WHO) declared the world SARS-free, the disease had spread to 29 countries, resulting in 8096 probable cases and 774 deaths worldwide, and significant social and economic impacts in areas with sustained transmission. Similarly, air transport played a key role in the global spread of influenza H1N1 (also known as 'swine flu'), with confirmed cases in at least 171 countries during the first few months of the 2009 pandemic (Khan et al. 2009).

Ongoing changes in the production and global trade of food also have important public health implications. The growing demand for meat products has led to an intensification of livestock production in many regions and a dramatic increase in the quantity of meat transported around the world for both processing and trade. This trend has the potential to affect infectious disease risk in different ways (Liverani et al. 2013). First, the quantitative increase in production and circulation of live and processed animals has enhanced the opportunities for transmission of viral infections and bacterial contaminants across livestock, wildlife, and humans. Second, intensification has involved a qualitative change in modes of livestock production, which may create favourable conditions for the emergence and dissemination of infectious diseases originating in animals. While modern production systems may be more isolated from contact with external sources of pathogens, their capacity to spread these diseases is considerable, through the concentration of large number of animals in communal housing, through the intensive movement of stock and feed, and through the extensive animal-based food value chains which they supply. Furthermore, the scale of livestock production is now global, with the international movement of livestock and animal products, and this is moving diseases more frequently and rapidly between countries, as we have seen in the recent outbreaks of livestock diseases that are transmissible to humans, like highly pathogenic avian influenza H5N1 (Coker et al. 2011). Similar trends can be observed in food-borne infections caused by contaminated fruits, vegetables or milk products. For example, recent outbreaks of *Salmonella poona* infection in the United States resulted from eating imported cantaloupe from source farms in Mexico, where microbial contamination was probably caused by inadequate hygiene and sanitation practices (CDC 2002).

Globalization has impacted on communicable disease in many ways, including through greater movement of goods, animals, and people. Economic globalization has brought benefits, wealth, and opportunities for many people, but has left many others in disadvantaged conditions, and thus more vulnerable to infections. For example, it is now clear that the abrupt transition of Russia to global capitalism after the end of the Soviet Union, and the resulting collapse of the health system, have largely contributed to the explosion of tuberculosis in this country from the early 1990s, while the incomplete antibiotic courses many patients received caused drug resistance (Coker et al. 2008). Poverty, inadequate hygiene and sanitation, employment insecurity, and lack of prospects are all key factors that can greatly amplify both the health and economic burden of infectious diseases. Links between the negative effects of globalization and the magnitude of the HIV/AIDS epidemic in Africa have been well documented (Barnett and Whiteside 2002). Evidence indicates that malaria and poverty are also connected. Although malaria transmission is determined by climate features and ecology, inadequate access to prevention methods such as bed-nets or repellents, weak health systems, lack of funding for government control programmes, and sub-standard housing are likely to enhance significantly the risk of infection (Whitty et al. 2008; Yeung et al. 2008).

Finally, globalization has led to changed patterns of food production and agriculture, including significant changes in land use and the environment that may affect the emergence and spread of infections in complex ways. Man-made interventions such as deforestation and urbanization alter fundamental ecosystems and the geographical distribution of human populations and animal species, with mixed effects that may increase or reduce the risk of infectious disease emergence, re-emergence or transmission (Fornace et al. 2013). Urban growth has the potential to reduce vector-borne diseases by disrupting the ecosystem of some vectors, but can create new opportunities for others. In many cities, for example, widespread stagnant water (e.g. in flower vases, buckets, and discarded tyres) provides ideal breeding sites for *Aedis aegyptis* mosquitoes, which can spread dengue fever to humans (Saker et al. 2007). Disease risk is further enhanced where the high mobility of urban dwellers and commuters has the potential to spread pathogens between different areas of the city and between different cities.

✎ **Activity 12.1**

Access the website of Health Map (www.healthmap.org), a freely available online system for disease outbreak monitoring and real-time surveillance of emerging public health threats. Identify a recent disease outbreak in your country or another country. Can you tell whether and to what extent the outbreak can be associated with globalization?

Feedback

> You should first clarify whether the disease spreads by direct transmission (from one host to another host) or indirect transmission (from host to host by means of a vector, such as the mosquito). You should then consider the context in which the outbreak occurred, including changes that may have affected host or vector behaviour (such as travel or urbanization), changes in the pathogen (such as mutations leading to antimicrobial resistance or increased virulence), and their interactions (such as lack of adequate prevention measures).

The globalization of infectious disease prevention and control

From the International Sanitary Conferences to the WHO

Globalizing processes and increasing mobility of people and goods have created new opportunities for the emergence and transnational spread of infectious agents. At the same time, the intensification of international relations and exchanges has led to the development of new institutional frameworks and cooperative arrangements to respond to these challenges.

Early efforts date back to the mid-nineteenth century, when national authorities began to attend international meetings to discuss the need for standard regulations and procedures against the rapid spread of diseases across countries. Since the plague pandemic in the fourteenth century, quarantine had been a standard practice for infectious disease control at ports and harbours, requiring ships coming from suspected or infected sites to remain at anchor for a month before docking. With the expansion of international trade in the nineteenth century, however, the mercantile elite increasingly contested old-fashioned quarantine measures, as they created costly delays to commercial traffic. In addition, the lack of international regulations was seen to undermine disease control efforts, given the inconsistency of sanitary measures across sea ports.

Driven by these concerns, in 1851 the delegates of twelve European states convened in Paris at the first International Sanitary Conference to agree on common quarantine measures against the spread of cholera, plague, and yellow fever. Despite six months of negotiations, the conference failed to reach an agreement, partly due to diverging opinions about both the cause and mode of transmission of cholera. Nonetheless, this event established a new institutional forum for international cooperation and dialogue in this area, which was further consolidated in subsequent meetings and negotiations.

After several failed attempts, the first International Sanitary Convention was finally approved in 1892, to establish quarantine regulations for ships travelling through the Suez Canal. Opened in 1861, the canal was a key transportation route for international trade. However, medical administrators were concerned that the canal might be a channel for the spread in Europe of health threats that were perceived to originate in Asia and the Middle East. Similar concerns about the need to protect the European space from 'Asiatic' diseases were reflected in subsequent sanitary agreements, such as those regulating the flow of people during the annual Mecca pilgrimage (Huber 2006).

Over the following decades, international conferences became a regular forum for health authorities and researchers, leading to the adoption of additional treaties on specific problems. Further developments included the establishment of the Pan-American Sanitary Bureau in Washington in 1896 and the *Office International d'Hygiène Publique* (OIHP) in

Paris in 1907, both responsible for gathering information related to infectious disease outbreaks. Of particular importance was the public health work of the League of Nations (1919), whose administrative structure with three bodies (General Advisory Health Council, Health Committee, and Secretariat) was a precursor to the World Health Organization. While the primary aim of the League of Nations was the promotion of collective security and the peaceful resolution of conflicts, member states were also required 'to take steps in matters of international concern for the prevention and control of disease', including sharing of epidemiological data and the standardization of biological products.

At the end of the Second World War, these pioneering efforts in international health cooperation were carried on by the United Nations and its health agency, the World Health Organization (WHO). Established in 1948, the WHO incorporated into a single body the former international health offices, including the Pan-American Sanitary Bureau, the League of Nations Health Organization, the *Office International d'Hygiène Publique*, and the *Conseil Sanitaire, Maritime et Quarantenaire* in Alexandria, Egypt. In addition, the WHO was given the mandate to unify the patchwork of *ad hoc* sanitary conventions into a single set of binding rules on quarantine requirements, called the International Sanitary Regulations (ISR). Under the ISR (1951), WHO member states were mandated to notify outbreaks of 'quarantinable' diseases (plague, cholera, smallpox, yellow fever, typhus, and relapsing fever), and to provide supplementary information on 'the source and type of the disease, the number of cases and deaths, the conditions affecting the spread of the diseases, and the prophylactic measures taken' (WHO 1951).

Similar to early agreements, these rules reflected the tension between public health and the imperative of global trade, namely the need to 'ensure the maximum security against the international spread of disease with the minimum interference with world traffic' (WHO 1951). Yet, the new regime of international health cooperation was different on fundamental grounds. Whereas previous interventions were underscored by the commercial interests of colonial powers and the need to protect the European space from external threats, the mandate of the WHO was supported by a universal vision of human health and well-being (Liverani and Coker 2012). Indeed, the preamble of the WHO Constitution (1948) states that 'the enjoyment of the highest attainable standard of health is one of the fundamental rights of every human being without distinction of race, religion, political belief, economic or social condition' (WHO 1948). Furthermore, the new legal framework granted equal sovereign rights to newly independent states and former colonial powers. Whereas colonial administrators controlled and distributed internationally reports of disease outbreaks through dedicated offices (such as the Far Eastern Bureau of the League of Nations, located in Singapore), under the ISR all WHO member states had legal control of epidemiological information.

In addition to the administration of international treaties and collection of epidemiological data, since its foundation the WHO has conducted many other activities for communicable disease prevention and control, including the development of international guidelines and the coordination of campaigns on global diseases. The campaign for the eradication of smallpox (1966–80) is often credited as one of the most important achievements of the WHO to date. Based on a combination of global surveillance, prevention measures, and vaccination programmes, the campaign successfully ended the transmission of a disease that caused about 300 million deaths in the twentieth century alone, largely in low- and middle-income countries. Other WHO campaigns on global diseases, however, have been far less successful. For example, malaria control and elimination programmes have repeatedly fallen below expectations, highlighting the many technical and institutional challenges involved in the WHO's ambitious mandate to improve health worldwide (Lee 2008).

Institutional change and global initiatives

During the 1970s, success in reducing the incidence of infectious disease in high-income countries led to complacency about the need for sustained prevention and control measures. In 1967, the Surgeon General of the United States, William Stewart, stated: 'The time has come to close the book on infectious diseases. We have basically wiped out infection in the United States' (Upshur 2008). It was anticipated that developing countries would also undergo a similar epidemiological transition from infectious to non-communicable disease burden, ushered in by the development of new vaccines and technologies.

From the 1980s, however, the dramatic rise of malaria cases in the Global South, the emergence of new problems such as multi-drug resistant tuberculosis, and the global impact of the HIV/AIDS pandemic brought renewed emphasis on the importance of infectious disease control. Furthermore, the complexity of socio-economic challenges associated with these diseases required novel approaches and institutional arrangements, and the active role of new actors beyond governments and established international agreements.

The case of HIV/AIDS illustrates the nature of these changes. During the 1980s, the direction of early international efforts against HIV/AIDS was mainly a responsibility of the WHO, which developed a Special Programme on AIDS and a global strategy to coordinate national policies and the adoption of common guidelines. However, it soon became apparent that the magnitude and complexity of the disease required the institutional support of a wider range of organizations. As a result, other specialized agencies of the United Nations became actively involved in the global campaign against HIV/AIDS, including UNDP, UNFPA, UNICEF, UNESCO, the World Bank, and FAO, providing input in their specific areas of expertise. For example, over the past decade, UNICEF has developed several programmes on mother-to-child transmission, expanding access to treatment for pregnant and breastfeeding women living with HIV. The World Bank has also become a prominent institutional actor in HIV/AIDS campaigns, partly in recognition of the link between disease burden and economic development (Lee 2008). In addition, a new UN programme, UNAIDS, was created to coordinate and support global action against the pandemic.

In parallel with these institutional developments, global responses to HIV/AIDS and other infectious diseases have increasingly been implemented through radically new cooperative arrangements, which have brought new actors and resources to improve health outcomes in developing countries. Some examples of these 'global health partnerships' are the Global Fund to fight AIDS, Tuberculosis and Malaria (the Global Fund), the World Bank's Multi-country AIDS Programme (MAP), and the GAVI Alliance on immunization. While these initiatives have been driven by different goals and approaches, they are all characterized by the involvement of multiple stakeholders in both decision-making and the delivery of health interventions, including national governments, non-governmental organizations (NGOs), pharmaceutical companies, and private foundations such as the Bill and Melinda Gates Foundation. Managers of global health partnerships have typically invested considerable resources in advocacy and communication campaigns, leading to a significant increase in aid funds and donor commitments. As a result, the health sector in many developing countries has received an unprecedented level of support, which enabled a substantial scaling up of treatment, prevention, and care services. Despite many positive outcomes, however, concerns have been raised about some downsides that global health providers may have on national health systems. Critics have argued that the focus on 'high-profile' infectious diseases may divert resources and attention from other important public health problems, which are not covered by funded programmes. In addition, there are key issues of sustainability; funding is usually given on an *ad hoc* basis to implement multi-annual programmes, but there are no mechanisms to ensure continued support in the long term (see Chapter 7).

Infectious disease control is also affected by antimicrobial and viral resistance (AMR), which has become an increasingly important issue globally. While resistance to antimicrobials is a natural process, many fewer new antimicrobials are in the pipeline at a time when many organisms have acquired multiple resistance to antimicrobials, such as, for example, multi-drug resistant tuberculosis (MDR-TB). Antimicrobial and viral resistance is posing a real and increasing challenge to the control of infectious diseases (Smith and Coast 2013).

The new system of global surveillance

As discussed, the post-Second World War regime of global disease surveillance was based on a set of binding rules, the International Sanitary Regulations, under which signatory states were mandated to notify the WHO about outbreaks of specific diseases and maintain adequate public health structures at key entry/exit points (e.g. sea ports and airports). This approach was largely derived from the early sanitary conventions of the nineteenth century and remained stagnant for many years. The only significant changes until recently included the removal of the provisions related to the annual pilgrimage to Mecca, the renaming of the ISR as International Health Regulations (IHR) in 1969, and changes in the list of diseases, as occurred when smallpox was removed in 1981 after eradication (Fidler 2005). From the late 1980s, however, it became increasingly apparent that this regulatory framework was insufficient to keep up with the pressure of globalization and resulting health challenges. First, with the compression of travelling times by air transport, the application of quarantine measures to suspected or confirmed cases was inadequate to control the transnational spread of diseases; people could contract a disease in one country, and cross borders by air travel within the incubation period well before the appearance of any symptoms. Second, despite the binding nature of the IHR, WHO member states repeatedly failed to comply with the obligations of notification, for example, due to fears of economic losses that may result from disruptions to trade and tourism. Last but not least, the focus of legal provisions on a short list of known diseases became, anachronistic in the new context of global public health, characterized by an increasing emphasis on the *potential* threats of novel or evolving pathogens, as captured in the concept of *emerging infectious diseases*. Fashioned in the USA in the late 1980s, this concept has had an active role in shaping public health approaches worldwide by stressing the impact of globalizing processes on rapid microbial change and adaptation, and the resulting need for constant surveillance of potential infections (Weir and Mykhalovskiy 2009). In the aftermath of recent public health crises associated with previously unknown diseases such as severe acute respiratory syndrome (SARS), bovine spongiform encephalopathy (BSE), Nipah virus, and avian influenza H5N1, global monitoring of emerging infections has become a priority on the agenda of health policy-makers.

 Activity 12.2

Browse the Internet and locate news reports about highly pathogenic avian influenza H5N1, a viral disease that originates in animal sources and can cause severe illness and death in humans. Do the reports discuss the implications of H5N1 for national economies? Is there any consideration of the global impact of the disease?

Feedback

You may have found reports of individual cases of patients, or news coverage discussing symptoms. Rarely do these articles discuss the economic implications. However, they often highlight the risks arising from the H5N1 on the basis of one individual case. Reading such coverage, we can envisage the effect that might have on the economy, with tourists avoiding travel to an area where a case is reported, and trade being adversely affected.

In the context of increased attention to emerging infectious diseases, the WHO undertook a major revision of international agreements, which led to the adoption of the new International Health Regulations in 2005. By contrast with former provisions, the focus of surveillance shifted from a limited number of specific diseases to *any* events that might constitute a public health threat of international concern, including unknown diseases, as well as the accidental or deliberate spread of nuclear, chemical, and biological contaminants. Another important innovation was the recognition of unofficial information sources (such as online news and social media) as a key component of the surveillance system, allowing the WHO to set forth recommendations based on such information, even in the absence of cooperation or agreement from affected member states. This is to avoid delay in reporting by member states where these may fear negative economic consequences, especially as there is no mechanism to compensate for loss of economic activity.

In practice, the new strategy relies on the operations of *early warning systems*, which help detect disease outbreaks or other health threats through constant monitoring of Internet media and international news, or reports from volunteers worldwide. For example, the Global Public Health Intelligence Network (GPHIN), developed by Canada's Public Health Agency, scans Internet media in nine languages through automated strategies to identify any messages that may suggest the occurrence of outbreaks. Given the unofficial nature of such sources, the WHO's Global Alert and Response (GAR) team is mandated to verify the validity of the report and perform risk analysis through a sequence of procedures, including initial verification through contacts from WHO regional offices, national authorities, and additional sources, and an evaluation of the potential for international spread. If the incoming report meets the required criteria for a public health event of international concern, the WHO is responsible for the dissemination of official alerts to national and international authorities and the Global Outbreak Alert and Response Network (GOARN), and the development of an action plan for the coordination of international response.

✎ **Activity 12.3**

Access again the website of Health Map (www.healthmap.org), and identify another recent disease outbreak in your country or another country. Health Map provides epidemiological intelligence by automatically aggregating disparate data sources, including online news, eyewitness reports, social media, and reports from NGOs working in the field. If you were a public health expert working in the WHO's Global Alert Response team, what would you do to verify the outbreak information?

Feedback

Outbreak verification involves a sequence of practices, which are aimed at evaluating the validity and potential threat of the reported information. You should first evaluate the nature of the infection and the potential to spread across borders, its geographical context, and the country's capacity to respond, as well as the reliability of the information source. You should then seek confirmation of details from health authorities in the countries concerned, usually through the WHO representative, and possibly also unofficial sources working in the field, such as the International Red Cross or NGOs.

The WHO-coordinated system of global surveillance and response is not the only system operating today; other event-based global systems have been developed under different arrangements and responsibilities, including MedISys (run by the Health Threats Unit at the Directorate General of Health and Consumer Affairs of the European Commission), Argus (funded by the US, and based at the Georgetown University Medical Center), Biocaster (based at the National Institute of Informatics in Tokyo), and Health Map (funded by Google, Inc., and located at the Harvard Medical School). In addition, disease surveillance networks have also been established at the regional level, such as the European Surveillance System (TESSy), based at the European Centre for Disease Prevention and Control, and the Mekong Basin Disease Surveillance (MBDS) network in Southeast Asia. In this fragmented context, the WHO has developed plans to establish a 'network of networks', linking together existing local, regional, national, and international networks. However, questions remain about the feasibility of such a 'super-surveillance system', as this will involve considerable coordination of efforts and the solution of complex technical problems.

Summary

Globalization has posed unprecedented challenges to public health. Increases in mobility of people have facilitated the rapid spread of communicable diseases across countries, while changes in food production systems have created new interactions between humans and animals, which have the potential to promote the emergence and spread of new diseases. At the same time, new technologies and the intensification of international relations have created opportunities to address these threats. Furthermore, the establishment of new cooperative arrangements, such as global health partnerships, has contributed to strengthening capacities for infectious disease control in developing countries, where interventions are most needed. Yet, key challenges remain. The emergence of new influential actors in the increasingly crowded field of global public health has brought additional resources and innovative approaches to infectious disease control, but has also resulted in the fragmentation of global health action, poor coordination, and duplication of efforts. Most importantly, many of the benefits derived from economic globalization have disproportionately accrued to wealthy countries, leaving poor nations more vulnerable to the burden of infectious diseases. Inequitable access to resources for the prevention, treatment, and control of infectious diseases is arguably the most important challenge ahead, requiring continued investments and innovative approaches in policy responses.

References

Barnett, T. and Whiteside, A. (2002) *AIDS in the Twenty-first Century: Disease and Globalization*. Basingstoke: Palgrave Macmillan.

Briggs, A. (1961) Cholera and society in the nineteenth century, *Past and Present*, 19: 76–96.

Centers for Disease Prevention and Control (CDC) (2002) Multistate outbreaks of salmonella serotype poona infections associated with eating cantaloupe from Mexico – United States and Canada, 2000–2002, *Morbidity and Mortality Weekly Report*, 51 (46): 1044–7.

Coker, R.J., Atun, R. and McKee, M. (2008) *Health Systems and the Challenge of Communicable Diseases: Experiences from Europe and Latin America*. Maidenhead: Open University Press.

Coker, R.J., Hunter, B.M., Rudge, J.W., Liverani, M. and Hanvoravongchai, P. (2011) Emerging infectious diseases in southeast Asia: regional challenges to control, *The Lancet*, 377 (9765): 599–609.

Fidler, D.P. (2005) From international sanitary conventions to global health security: the new international health regulations, *Chinese Journal of International Law*, 4 (2): 325–92.

Fornace, K., Liverani, M., Rushton, J. and Coker, R.J. (2013) Effects of land use changes and agricultural practices on the emergence and re-emergence of human viral diseases, in S. Singh (ed.) *Viral Infections and Global Change*. Hoboken, NJ: Wiley-Blackwell.

Gushulak, B.D. and MacPherson, D.W. (2006) The basic principles of migration health: population mobility and gaps in disease prevalence, *Emerging Themes in Epidemiology*, 3: 3.

Huber, V. (2006) The unification of the globe by disease? The international sanitary conferences on cholera, 1851–1894, *The Historical Journal*, 49: 453–76.

International Civil Aviation Organization (ICAO) (2014) *The World of Civil Aviation: Facts and Figures* [http://www.icao.int/sustainability/Pages/FactsFigures.aspx; accessed 25 February 2014].

Khan, K., Arino, J., Hu, W., Raposo, P., Sears, J., Calderon, F. et al. (2009) Spread of a novel influenza A (H1N1) virus via global airline transportation, *New England Journal of Medicine*, 361 (2): 212–14.

Lee, K. (2008) *The World Health Organization (WHO)*. London: Routledge.

Liverani, M. and Coker, R. (2012) Protecting Europe from diseases: from the international sanitary conferences to the ECDC, *Journal of Health Politics, Policy, and Law*, 37 (6): 915–34.

Liverani, M., Waage, J., Barnett, T., Pfeiffer, D.U., Rushton, J., Rudge, J.W. et al. (2013) Understanding and managing zoonotic risk in the new livestock industries. *Environmental Health Perspectives*, 121 (8): 873–7.

Ruan, S., Wang, W. and Lewin, S. (2006) The effect of global travel on the spread of SARS, *Mathematical Biosciences and Engineering*, 3 (1): 205–18.

Saker, L., Lee, K. and Cannito, B. (2007) Infectious disease in the age of globalization, in I. Kawachi and S. Wamala (eds.) *Globalization and Health*. Oxford: Oxford University Press.

Smith, R. and Coast, E. (2013) The true cost of antimicrobial resistance, *British Medical Journal*, 346: f1493.

Upshur, R. (2008) Ethics and infectious disease, *Bulletin of the World Health Organization*, 86 (8): 654.

Weir, L. and Mykhalovskiy, E. (2009) *Global Public Health Vigilance: Creating a World on Alert*. London: Routledge.

Whitty, C.J., Chandler, C., Ansah, E., Leslie, T. and Staedke, S.G. (2008) Deployment of ACT antimalarials for treatment of malaria: challenges and opportunities, *Malaria Journal*, 7 (suppl. 1): S7.

WHO (1948) *Constitution of the World Health Organization*. Geneva: World Health Organization.

WHO (1951) *International Sanitary Regulations*. Geneva: World Health Organization.

Yeung, S., Van Damme, W., Socheat, D., White, N.J. and Mills, A. (2008) Access to artemisinin combination therapy for malaria in remote areas of Cambodia, *Malaria Journal*, 7: 96.

Globalization, environmental change, and impacts on human health

13

Carolyn Stephens and Tony McMichael

Overview

In this chapter, you will explore the impacts of globalization on global environmental change (GEC) and its related effects on human health. You will begin by examining GEC, how it relates to globalization (a mix of economic, social, cultural, technological, physical, and other changes), and the sorts of health impacts GEC might have, both now and in future. You will examine specific examples of research in relation to global environmental changes and health, and consider your own impact on GEC.

Learning objectives

After working through this chapter, you will be able to:

- distinguish global environmental change (GEC) in general from more traditional environmental hazards
- understand how GEC relates to globalization
- recognize the ways in which GEC, directly and indirectly, affects human health
- understand some of the difficulties in estimating the health impacts of GEC

Key terms

Adaptation: An action (or spontaneous change) that lessens the adverse impacts of GEC.

Biodiversity: The natural range of species (or intra-species genetic strains) within an ecosystem that provides a source of resilience, stability, and productivity.

Carrying capacity: The size of population that can be indefinitely supported by the natural resource base of the specified geographic area.

Climate change: Long-term change (over decades, centuries or millennia) in average meteorological conditions (such as temperature and rainfall).

Climate variability: Shifts in climatic patterns that are relatively short term (over months to years) and that go beyond individual weather events.

Ecosystem: The complex of a community of organisms and its environment functioning as an ecological unit.

Extreme weather events: Extreme transient weather conditions, which differ from longer-term conditions that define a prevailing *climate*.

Global environmental change: Large-scale human-induced changes in the Earth's natural environment in recent decades as a reflection of unprecedented impacts on the biosphere.

Scenario: A description of a set of conditions, now or, plausibly, in the future.

Understanding global environmental change

Humans (like other species) depend upon the world's complex geophysical and ecological systems to sustain their health and survival. This natural environment not only provides air, food, and water, it also provides a range of life-supporting environmental 'goods' (e.g. clothing materials, shelter, and energy) and 'services' (e.g. constancy of local climate, pollination of food plants, and the uptake of carbon dioxide and production of oxygen via plant photosynthesis).

Over many millennia, human societies have found ways to increase the 'carrying capacity' of their local environment by exploiting local resources, modifying the ecosystem, and supplementing local food supplies and other materials via trade. This (in the shorter term) has been a triumph of human culture. Human societies have moved from a hunter-gatherer existence, to agrarianism (coupled increasingly with urban living), then to industrialization, and today to a post-industrial 'information age'. Each such change has required a trade-off between the resultant increase in human population density (via gains in environmental carrying capacity), and longer-term weakening of the local environment's life-supporting capacity (McMichael 2005; UNEP-GEAS 2012; WRI/UNDP/World Bank 2005).

The historical record suggests that failure to maintain the natural environmental resource base has been a recurring cause of societal instability, decline, and collapse. Overuse and degradation of freshwater supplies have been a particularly important problem. A well-known example is Easter Island in the southeast Pacific. The Polynesian people, who settled on the previously uninhabited island around AD 900, initially thrived. However, they eventually denuded the island's forest, which led to massive soil erosion, loss of wood for canoes for fishing, and the extinction of pollinating birds. Their numbers dwindled, conditions deteriorated, and warfare and cannibalism broke out. When Dutch explorers landed in 1722 there were fewer than 2000 inhabitants. By around 1850, the survivors had dwindled to a few hundred. Equally, the Mayan civilization appears to have collapsed, around 1000 years ago, under the dual stress of an adverse climatic cycle over several centuries and excessive agricultural demand on freshwater supplies.

Contemporary global environmental change

During the past two centuries, human impact on the environment has increased dramatically. Populations expanded approximately eight-fold and the material-intensity and energy-intensity of economic activity greatly increased. The world's population, currently 7 billion, is expected to reach 9 billion by 2050. The total human 'carrying capacity' of Earth is neither fixed nor certain, and depends on future patterns of consumption and waste generation (UNEP-GEAS 2012). Today, we face unfamiliar problems posed by global environmental change. The best known is global climate change, occurring in response to the excessive emission of greenhouse gases into the lower atmosphere, especially the release of carbon dioxide from fossil fuel combustion.

An estimation from the Fifth Assessment Report (2013) of the International Panel on Climate Change (IPCC), based on multiple independent datasets, shows that the globally averaged combined land and ocean surface temperature data (as calculated by a fitted linear trend) show a warming of 0.85°C [0.65 to 1.06] over the period 1880 to 2012. The total increase between the average of the 1850–1900 period and the 2003–2012 period is 0.78°C [0.72 to 0.85], based on the single longest dataset available (Stocker et al. 2013). According to the World Resources Institute, total global emissions grew 12.7 per cent between 2000 and 2005, an average of 2.4 per cent a year. However, individual sectors grew at rates between 40 per cent and near zero, and there are substantial differences in sectoral growth rates between developed and developing countries. Figure 13.1 summarizes contributions of different sectors to carbon emissions in 2005 (WRI/UNDP/ World Bank 2005).

Other global environmental changes include:

- human-induced changes to the middle atmosphere (stratosphere) resulting in depletion of (ultraviolet-shielding) stratospheric ozone;
- changes to global elemental cycles (nitrogen, phosphorus, sulphur, carbon, etc.);
- biodiversity impacts:
  - loss/extinction of species,
  - redistribution of species (invasion);
- changes to food-producing ecosystems:
  - land cover, loss of soil fertility,
  - coastal and marine ecosystems (including fisheries);
- desertification;
- changes to the hydrological cycle, and depletion of freshwater supplies including major underground aquifers;
- worldwide dissemination of persistent organic pollutants (POPs);
- urbanization (e.g. land-use, pressure on regional ecosystems, massive waste generation).

Human alteration of Earth and its 'operating system', including on a global scale (historically unprecedented), is now substantial and growing. Between one-third and one-half of the land surface has been transformed by human action; the carbon dioxide concentration in the atmosphere has increased by a little over 40 per cent since the beginning of the Industrial Revolution; more atmospheric nitrogen is 'fixed' as biologically activated nitrogen by humanity than by all natural terrestrial sources combined; more than half of all accessible surface fresh water is put to use by humanity; and about one-quarter of the bird species on Earth have been driven to extinction as part of an ongoing and very rapid human-driven extinction crisis – 'The Sixth Extinction'.

By these and other standards, scientists are now describing the human population as a 'global geo-physical force', affecting the planet and its functioning in unprecedented

World Greenhouse Gas Emissions in 2005
Total:44,153 MtCO eq.

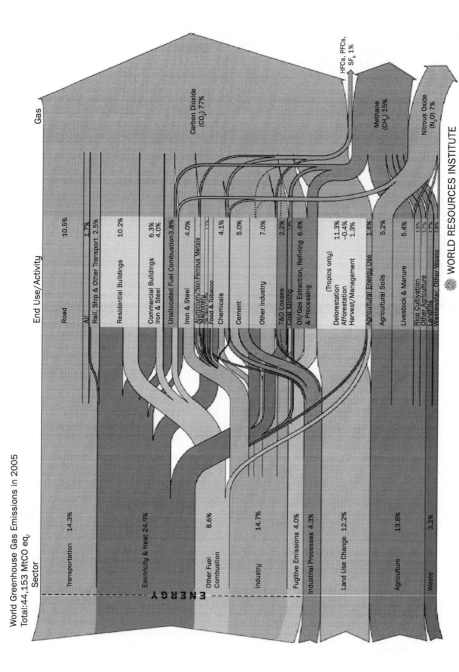

Figure 13.1 World greenhouse gas emissions by sector and activity, 2005

Source: WRI (2013)

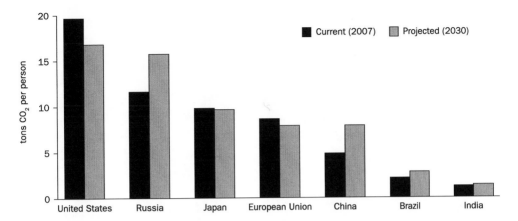

Figure 13.2 Carbon emissions by country, 2007 and projected, 2030 (tonnes CO_2 per capita)

Source: WRI (2013)

ways (UNEP-GEAS 2012). There is serious international consideration of calling this age of human domination and its disruptions of planetary resources and functioning *The Anthropocene* – to follow the 11,000-year climatically stable and warmer Holocene that emerged after the last cold glacial period ('ice age').

To understand better the nature of global environmental changes, consider the world's carbon cycle. Carbon, the basis of life on Earth, circulates continuously between air, vegetation, soil, and oceans. Meanwhile, vast and essentially immobile stores of carbon sit underground in ancient fossilized deposits of coal, oil, and methane gas, and under the oceans as limestone sediment. Alongside the several hundred billion tonnes of carbon that circulate naturally through the biosphere each year, humans, globally averaged, now annually release to the atmosphere approximately 14 extra tonnes of carbon per person – a human-generated total of around 9 billion tonnes per year. And, as a 2012 UNEP report states, 'we are not a single person; we are now seven billion people and we are adding one million more people roughly every 4.8 days' (UNEP-GEAS 2012).

The distribution of national per-person carbon dioxide emissions is very uneven. [Note that the ratio of molecular weight for carbon dioxide versus carbon is 44:12 – one tonne of oxidized carbon yields 3.7 tonnes of carbon dioxide.] Figure 13.2 shows national per-capita carbon dioxide emissions figures for 2007 and predicted for 2030 – and shows that in 2007 people living in the United States contributed around 19 tonnes per year while the figure in India remained at just over 1 tonne. As the new and expanding economies of Brazil, Russia, India, and China (the so-called BRIC countries) increase their carbon dioxide outputs, outputs from Europe and North America are anticipated to decrease. Around half of this extra atmospheric carbon dioxide is absorbed by Earth's natural 'sinks' (oceans, forests, and soils). However, the rest (4–5 billion tonnes) accumulates in the lower atmosphere as extra carbon dioxide, which changes the heat-trapping capacity of the lower atmosphere and thus warms the Earth's surface.

Relationship of global environmental changes to globalization

Globalization describes the scale and connectedness of our economic, technological, cultural, and other activities. At first sight, there seems to be a close *negative* connection

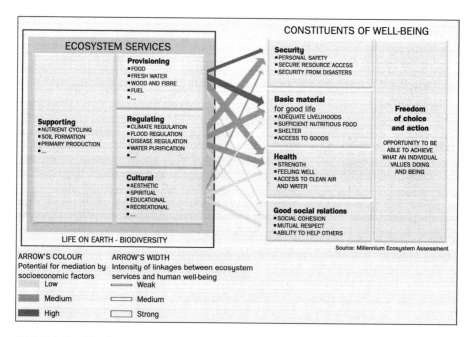

Figure 13.3 Relationships between human populations and their economic and social activities, and the resultant links of the ecosystem with human health and activities

Source: Millennium Assessment Report (2000)

between globalization and large-scale environmental change. For example, as urbanization and industrialization spread, they are linked to increased consumption patterns. As consumption increases, particularly of energy-intensive products such as cars, heating and cooling mechanisms, the emission of greenhouse gases increases. Yet we also seek a 'sustainable' future world, which will presumably be a globalized world – where we would work together to protect the planet and its resources.

In recent years, the United Nations has accorded increasing recognition and importance to 'ecosystem services' for human health and well-being, especially via the huge international scientific effort around the turn of the century that constituted the Millennium Ecosystem Assessment. Figure 13.3 shows the relationships between human populations and their economic and social activities, and the resultant links of the ecosystem with human health and activities (UNEP-WCMC 2011).

✎ **Activity 13.1**

1 List four ways in which globalization is likely to contribute to the occurrence of global changes to our ecosystem services.
2 Name four key changes in technology or human practice that would render a future globalized world more ecologically sustainable.

Feedback

1   Globalization might contribute to global environmental change and affect our ecosystem service in the following ways:

- Long-distance and rapid trade accelerates the inadvertent global distribution of
  'exotic' species of insects, animals, and plants. Some thrive in their new environments, disrupting ecosystems and displacing local food species.
- The intensification and increased corporate-control of world food production
  entail increasing use of energy and nitrogenous fertilizer. This has hugely
  increased the entry of activated nitrogenous compounds into the environment,
  changing the global nitrogen cycle, and causing significantly altered chemical
  balance and acidity in waterways and soils.
- As Chapter 12 highlights, the globalization of diets (in conjunction with rapid
  urbanization) stimulates demand for (excessive) meat consumption. This entails
  inefficient use of cereal grain as animal feed, and exerts great physical and
  chemical pressures on land and water resources. This includes deforestation
  to open up pastoral land. Widespread environmental degradation and carbon
  dioxide emissions result.
- As trade intensifies and spreads, many countries are driven to develop exports
  to generate foreign exchange. In exploiting their distinctive export opportunities, they may do so in ways that damage the local natural resource base. The
  widespread occurrence of uncontrolled logging is a well-known example, leading
  to widespread loss of locally valued forest products, species extinctions, flood
  control, mobilization of infectious agents (especially viruses) into human communities, and release of greenhouse gases.

2   Examples of technological and behavioural changes facilitating 'sustainability' are:

- De-carbonizing our energy generation (e.g. use of renewables such as wind
  power, nuclear energy, development of 'clean coal' technology).
- Reducing energy demands via public transport, energy-efficient domestic products, improved housing design.
- Laws that require imported (especially luxury) foods to reflect their full environmental cost (e.g. exhaust gases from air-freighted wine and foods).
- Re-orienting diets towards naturally health-promoting and environmentally
  benign production sources: fresh fruit and vegetables, meat in moderation (and
  produced by less fat-intensive means), unrefined carbohydrate foods.
- Re-engineering industry, agriculture, and domestic/garden design to lessen the
  demand for fresh water; better technologies for the recycling of water.
- Controlled use of pesticides and herbicides, to minimize the (often long-term)
  damage to ecosystems and threatened extinction of species.

The risks to human health from global environmental change

The scale of GEC and its many different modes and paths of causal influence on health
outcomes represent an important difference from environmental concerns that relate to
localized toxicological or microbiological hazards. Indeed, these environmental changes

are manifestations of the 'ecological deficit' into which humans are forcing the planet. Humans are thus crossing a new frontier, and there is a need to understand the range of likely adverse health impacts and other consequences (Stocker et al. 2013).

First, we will consider the health risks of global climate change before looking at a range of the main known or anticipated health risks from other major categories of GEC.

The climate system and greenhouse gases

To date, the most extensive, and best developed, GEC-related health risk assessments have been done in relation to stratospheric ozone depletion (with its mostly direct-acting risks to skin and eyes) and global climate change. This section focuses on the latter – global climate change – an exemplar of global environmental change, and examines the methods of studying, and estimating, the resultant health impacts.

There remains debate about the relationship between human-generated 'greenhouse gases' and the world's climate system. Over the past decade, the number of doubters has declined steadily as the science of climate change has matured, and some early signs of the (non-human) impact of recent global warming have now emerged. We now know:

1 Various greenhouse gases, especially carbon dioxide and water vapour, occur naturally in the atmosphere. By capturing some of the solar energy reradiated outwards by the Earth, those greenhouse gases warm the Earth's surface by around 32°C. The physics of this process is well understood.
2 Over eons, the atmospheric concentration of greenhouse gases has varied in close correlation with the temperature of the Earth's surface.
3 Other factors affect the Earth's temperature, including variation in solar activity, the amount of volcanic activity, and (on longer time-scales) the tilt of the Earth's axis and shape of its orbit.

Given this scientific knowledge, and that atmospheric carbon dioxide concentration has risen 40 per cent since the beginning of the Industrial Revolution 200 years ago, scientists predict that the Earth's temperature will rise. It has in fact risen unusually fast over the past quarter of a century, and the temporal and spatial characteristics of this rise indicate that most has been due to the increasing concentration of greenhouse gases. Nevertheless, uncertainties remain about the future greenhouse gas-emitting behaviours of societies, how the complex climate system will respond to future changes in atmospheric composition, how feedback processes will operate, and whether there are critical thresholds that will cause abrupt climatic-environmental changes. Debate therefore continues about the projected actual trajectories of global temperature over the coming century (Grundmann 2006).

Naturally occurring greenhouse gases (including water vapour, carbon dioxide, nitrous oxide, methane, and ozone) comprise about 2 per cent of the atmosphere. The Earth's surface absorbs some solar radiation and re-radiates it outwards as long-wave (infrared) radiation. Some of this infrared radiation is absorbed by atmospheric greenhouse gases and re-radiated back to Earth, thus raising the average surface temperature to its present 15°C. Without this warming, the average temperature of the Earth would be about 33°C colder and permanently frozen over.

World average temperature and atmospheric carbon dioxide concentration have varied over the past millennia. These changes have been estimated from the Antarctic ice cores.

Earth's temperature has naturally varied within a range of 10°C, as the planet has moved in and out of global glaciations. It is against this background that humankind is now super-imposing additional carbon dioxide 'greenhouse forcing'. Most of the recent emissions have occurred during the twentieth century as a result of burgeoning economic activity. Currently, the rate of emission remains unabated as industrialization proceeds in the developing world with China, India, and Brazil becoming major emitters.

In its most recent, Fifth Assessment Report in 2013, the UN's Intergovernmental Panel on Climate Change forecast a rise in average world temperature of around 3–4°C by 2100, although there is necessarily uncertainty around this estimate since the behaviour of nations and their technologies cannot be foreseen. The warming would be (and is) greater at higher latitudes, especially in the northern hemisphere. This anticipated warming would be much more rapid than any natural warming experienced by humans since the advent of agriculture around 10,000 years ago. This extremely rapid rate of change will put many of the biosphere's ecosystems and species under stress.

There will also be regional changes in rainfall patterns, with increases over the oceans but reduction over much of the land surface, especially in various low-to-medium latitude mid-continental regions (central Spain, American mid-west, the Sahel, Amazonia), and in already arid areas in northwest India, the Middle East, northern Africa, and parts of Central America. Rainfall events will tend to intensify, with more frequent extreme events increasing the likelihood of flooding and droughts, as we are already witnessing in Europe and in Asia. Regional weather systems, including the great South-West Asian monsoon, could undergo latitudinal shift (Martens 2009).

Climatologists also anticipate that climate variability will increase with global climate change. Computer models and empirical evidence suggest there will be increasingly severe weather events, including more powerful storms and stronger winds, intensification of the El Niño cycle, and altered patterns of drought and rainfall. There is great inertia in the climate system. Even if the build-up in greenhouse gases is arrested by mid-century, the seas will continue to expand as the extra heat permeates the ocean and as on-land glaciers continue to melt at warmer temperature, rising by up to several metres over the coming thousand years.

With two-thirds of the world's population living within 60 km of the sea, a rise in sea level would have widespread health impacts. The countries most vulnerable to sea-level rise include Bangladesh and Egypt, with huge river delta farming populations, and Pakistan, Indonesia, and Thailand, with large coastal populations. Various low-lying small-island populations in the Pacific and Indian Oceans, with few material resources, face the prospect of wholesale displacement. A half-metre rise would approximately double the number (at today's population) who experience flooding annually from around 50 million to 100 million. Some of the world's coastal arable land and fish-nurturing mangroves would be damaged by sea-level rise. Rising seas would salinate coastal freshwater aquifers, particularly under small islands. A heightening of storm surges would damage coastal roadways, sanitation systems, and housing.

Health impacts of climate change

There are direct and indirect ways in which climate change can affect human health. Furthermore, some impacts will occur relatively immediately, while others will depend on a succession of changes in natural systems, and may occur incrementally. It should also be noted that there is, as yet, little empirical evidence that the process of climate *change* causes these health impacts. The anticipation and estimation of these health risks depend on extrapolation from the climate–health relationships previously observed within situations of natural climate variation and local trend. Hence, there is some debate as to when and where health impacts attributable to climate change *per se* might actually occur (Campbell-Lendrum and Corvalan 2007).

The anticipated direct health impacts include those due to changes in exposure to thermal extremes (heat and cold); increases in extreme weather events (floods, cyclones, storm-surges, droughts); and increased production of certain air pollutants and aero-allergens (spores and moulds). Decreases in winter mortality due to milder winters may compensate for increases in summer mortality due to the increased frequency of heatwaves.

Climate change, acting via less direct mechanisms, would affect regional food productivity. It would affect the transmission of many infectious diseases, especially water-, food-, and vector-borne diseases. Recent reports suggest that we may now be seeing some early impacts of climate change on infectious diseases. For example, tick-borne (viral) encephalitis in Sweden appears to have increased in response to a succession of warmer winters over the past two decades, and there is some (contentious) evidence of malaria ascending to higher altitudes in the eastern African highlands in association with local warming. In the longer term, these indirect impacts are likely to have greater magnitude than more direct impacts.

Vector-borne infections are of particular relevance. The distribution and abundance of vector organisms and intermediate hosts are affected by physical factors (temperature, precipitation, humidity, surface water, and wind) and biotic factors (vegetation, host species, predators, parasites, and human interventions). Modelling studies indicate that a temperature increase would cause net increases, worldwide, in the geographic range of various vector organisms, although some localized decreases might occur. Furthermore, temperature-related changes in the life cycle of both vector and pathogen (flukes, protozoa, bacteria, and viruses) would increase the potential transmission of many vector-borne diseases: malaria (mosquito), dengue (mosquito), and leishmaniasis (sand-fly), although schistosomiasis (water-snail) may undergo a net decrease (if water temperatures in many regions become too warm for the snail to thrive).

Modelling, allowing for future trends in trade and economic development, has been used to estimate the impacts of climate change on cereal grain yields (which account for 50–60 per cent of world food energy). The results indicate that a slight downturn is likely over the next half-century, but this would be greater in already food-insecure regions in South Asia, parts of Africa and Central America. Such downturns would increase the number of malnourished people by several tens of millions in the world. Figure 13.4 shows the alarming models for impacts of climate change on agricultural output.

Studies of the effect of climate change on food production show that yields of cereal grains are likely to decrease in the tropics where many countries are already under water stress. In particular, there is concern that climate change may increase the extent of malnutrition in Africa, and there is currently widespread evidence of undernutrition in countries of central, southern, and eastern Africa. Drought also leads to forest fires, which in some locations (especially Malaysia and Brazil) have been associated with an increased risk of respiratory disease, eye problems, injuries, and fatalities (Millar et al. 2007).

Of course, the health prospects are not all negative. Milder winters would reduce the seasonal winter-time mortality peak in temperate countries. A further increase in temperatures in currently hot regions might impair mosquito survival. Overall, however,

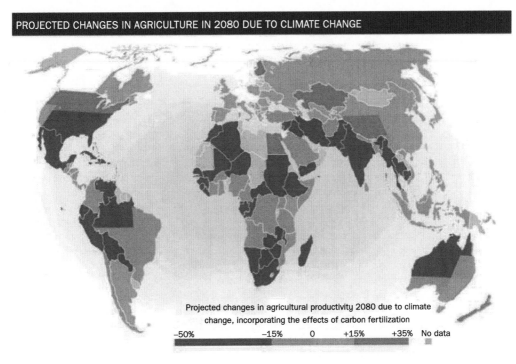

PROJECTED CHANGES IN AGRICULTURE IN 2080 DUE TO CLIMATE CHANGE

Projected changes in agricultural productivity 2080 due to climate
change, incorporating the effects of carbon fertilization

–50%   –15%   0   +15%   +35%   No data

Figure 13.4 Projected changes in agriculture in 2080 due to climate change

Source: Cline (2007)

scientists have consistently assessed that most climate change health impacts would be adverse in nature (Stocker et al. 2013).

As average surface temperatures gradually rise, an increase in climatic variability is likely. Indeed, the frequency and intensity of such events already appear to be increasing. Many scientists consider that human health and safety are more endangered by an impending increase in extreme and anomalous weather events than by changes in average climate conditions.

Increased variability of climate and extreme weather events

Not surprisingly, the prospect of extreme weather events also has triggered the concern of health experts (not just their imaginations), following an increase in devastating extreme events around the world, including heat waves, floods, and massive tropical storms (Stocker et al. 2013). The extent to which the severity of heat waves, and extreme events, fall outside of current distribution of weather is consistent with expectations of future climate change scenarios. Climatologists have long remarked that global warming will not simply manifest itself by a gradual climb in average temperatures. Rather, it is the frequency and intensity of extreme climatic events – such as heat waves, droughts, floods, and storms – that are expected to occur.

Extreme weather events such as severe storms, floods, and drought have claimed millions of lives since the turn of the century and have adversely affected the lives of many more as well as costing enormous amounts in property damage.

Degradation of the local environment can also contribute to vulnerability from flooding. For example, Hurricane Mitch, the most deadly hurricane to strike the western hemisphere in the past two centuries, caused 11,000 deaths and thousands of others were missing in Central America. Many fatalities occurred as a result of mudslides in deforested areas.

Although extreme weather variability impacts injuries, fatalities, and the incidence of diseases such as malaria, we must not lose sight of the myriad of other diseases and health outcomes affected by more subtle long-term climate change. Mosquito-borne diseases, such as dengue fever and encephalitis, are generally more influenced by ambient conditions than diseases passed directly from human to human. Formation of ozone air pollution is hastened by warmer temperatures and by the ongoing increase in rates of human-caused methane emissions. Excessive rainfall and runoff can lead to large numbers of microorganisms entering drinking water, and outbreaks of waterborne disease have been associated with heavy rainfall events in the United States and elsewhere.

Although the more dire scenarios of future climate change and its many disruptive and destructive consequences may be unlikely, the march of climate change still presents a formidable challenge for human population health, the health sector, and society as a whole. A tidal wave inundating a city is an easily identifiable disaster that, given enough warning, people may escape from. But most adverse health effects posed by climate change will occur via various and different complex pathways – and these will require interdisciplinary analyses and integrated prevention planning.

 Activity 13.2

1 What climate-related health events can you think of within the past 12 months, in your region of the world or elsewhere, that might illustrate the possibility of rapid changes in risks to health, or of 'surprise' impacts?
2 How easy/reasonable is it, at this stage, to attribute any such individual impact event to human-induced climate change?

Feedback

1 One example could be the extreme weather events that increased mortality significantly in some countries. This has included heat waves.
2 As you may have realized, it is difficult, which is why more research and monitoring are required.

In many cases, climate change is linked to other global environmental changes. The following sections outline some of the major health-related global environmental changes.

Stratospheric ozone depletion

Various human-produced industrial gases, especially halogenated compounds (such as the chlorofluorocarbons used for refrigeration and insulated packaging), destroy ozone molecules in the stratosphere. This allows greater penetration to the Earth's surface of solar ultraviolet radiation (UVR), particularly at higher (above approximately 35°) latitudes, including southern Australia, southern South America, Northern Europe, and Canada. This increase in UVR exposure, particularly shorter-wavelength UV-B, increases the risk of skin cancer (malignant melanoma, non-melanocytic cancers). Other risks include increases in the incidence of ocular cataracts, other eye disorders such as squamous-cell cancer of the conjunctiva, and suppression of the immune system (e.g. lower vaccination efficacy, reduced risk of autoimmune disorders).

Disruption and degradation of various ecosystems

The increasing human demand for space, materials, and food leads to increasingly rapid extinction of populations and species of plants and animals. This, in turn, can disrupt ecosystems that provide nature's goods and services. We may also lose, before discovery, many natural chemicals and genes with potential medical and health benefits (Alves and Rosa 2007; Myers et al. 2000). Meanwhile, 'invasive' species are spreading into new environments in association with intensified trade, population mobility, and food production. These bio-invasions have myriad consequences for health. For example, the spread of the water hyacinth in East Africa's Lake Victoria, introduced from Brazil as a decorative plant, has nurtured the water snails that transmit schistosomiasis and the proliferation of diarrhoeal disease organisms.

Impairment of food-producing ecosystems

Increasing pressures from agricultural and livestock production put stresses on arable lands and pastures. In the early twenty-first century, it is estimated one-third of the world's previously productive land is adversely affected by erosion, compaction, salinization, waterlogging, and chemicalization, which destroy organic content. Similar pressures on the world's ocean fisheries have left most severely depleted or stressed. There is also doubt whether there is an environmentally benign and socially acceptable way of using genetic engineering to increase food yields. Such yields are needed to produce sufficient food for another 3 billion persons over the next half century (Lawler 2009; McIntyre et al. 2010).

Loss of biodiversity

In November 2011, botanists on a remote island off Papua New Guinea discovered a new species of orchid – a uniquely and mysteriously night-flowering orchid. New to science, and with so much more to understand, this flower is threatened by deforestation (Stephens 2012). Also in November 2011, a survey of 583 conservation scientists reported an unanimous (99.5 per cent) view that '*it is likely a serious loss of biological diversity is underway at a global extent*' and that, for scientists, '*protection of biological diversity for its cultural and spiritual values and because of its usefulness to humans were low priorities, which suggests that many scientists do not fully support the utilitarian concept of ecosystem services'* (Rudd 2011). In terms of management, some scientists now advocate controversial conservation strategies such as triage (prioritization of species that provide unique or necessary functions to ecosystems) (Parr et al. 2009).

Meanwhile, there are many scientists who contend that there is an urgent need to improve understanding of the importance of biodiversity for human health and well-being, arguing that only an anthropocentric view of biodiversity within a paradigm 'ecosystem service' will enable decision-makers to prioritize the theme. A 2011 UN report argues that this need for understanding is especially urgent in fragile and vulnerable ecosystems where communities depend directly on the resources of their environment (UNEP-WCMC 2011).

It is generally accepted that the destruction of biodiverse ecosystems internationally is not by communities directly dependent on these ecosystems, but from processes such as deforestation, mining, resource extraction, and biopiracy, generated by external human demand. Rich countries and their populations are currently particularly responsible for the resource extraction that impacts negatively on biodiversity and on the well-being of local communities. However, increasingly, urban populations in every country demand resources and products from biodiverse regions, and with rising urban populations this threat is likely to increase.

Water stress

Freshwater supplies are coming under increasing pressure around the world (Figure 13.5). Various major (subterranean) aquifers, in all continents, are being depleted. In the world's mid-latitude belts, this is likely to be exacerbated by a decline in rainfall due to climate

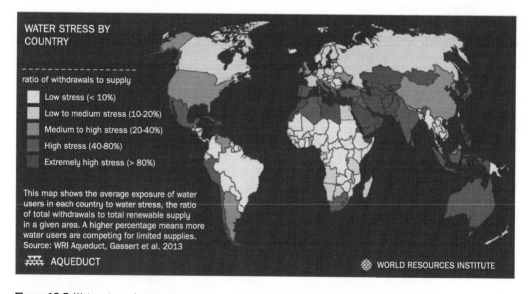

Figure 13.5 Water stress by country

Source: WRI (2013)

change – even as rainfall increases and becomes more intense at lower and higher latitudes. Agricultural and industrial demand, amplified by population growth, often greatly
exceeds both the rate of natural recharge of aquifers and flow rate within river systems.
Water-related political crises and even open conflict seem likely to occur in the near
future.

Summary: How do global environmental changes affect human health?

There are various pathways by which global environmental change can affect health.
Figure 13.6 illustrates three pathways of increasingly more complex and less direct character. At the top, there are examples of how changes in basic physical environmental
conditions (e.g. temperature extremes or level of ultraviolet irradiation) can directly affect
human biology and health. The other two pathways illustrate processes of increasing
complexity, including those that entail interactions between environmental conditions,
ecosystem functioning, and human social and economic conditions.

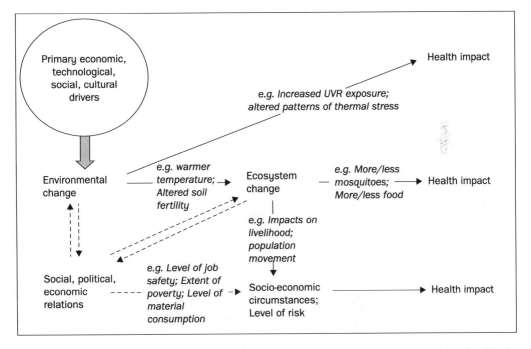

Figure 13.6 Main pathways by which global environmental changes can affect human population health. The
italicized items (on arrows) are for illustrative purposes only

✏ **Activity 13.3**

Fill in Table 13.1 (which shows eight types of global environmental change by eight categories of health risks) to indicate the known/likely strength of influence of each GEC on each health risk.

Table 13.1 Influence of eight types of global environmental change on eight health risks

	Physical injuries	Mental health impacts	Hunger and malnutrition	Infectious disease: VBDs	Infectious disease: Water- and food-borne	Cancers	Respiratory diseases	Cardio-vascular (heart blood vessels) diseases
Climate change				++				
Ozone depletion, and UVR exposure								
Freshwater depletion								
Soil degradation								
Biodiversity loss								
Damage to marine and coastal ecosystems								
Persistent organic pollutants (POPs)								
Urbanization and its impacts								

Use symbols to indicate very strong, (++), somewhat strong (+), possible (?), and no influence (0). If you think that climate change has a strong influence on the risk of vector-borne infectious diseases, put a ++ in that cell as shown.

Feedback

Your responses should look similar to those in Table 13.2.

Table 13.2 Influence of eight types of global environmental change on eight health risks (completed)

	Physical injuries	Mental health impacts	Hunger and malnutrition	Infectious disease: VBDs	Infectious disease: Water- and food-borne	Cancers	Respiratory diseases	Cardio-vascular (heart blood vessels) diseases
Climate change	+++	+	++	++	++	?	++	+
Ozone depletion, and UVR exposure	0	0	0	?	?	++	0	0
Freshwater depletion	0	+	+++	0	++	0	0	0
Soil degradation	0	?	+++	0	0	0	0	0
Biodiversity loss	0	++	+	+	0	+	0	?
Damage to marine and coastal ecosystems	0	0	+++	0	0	0	0	0
Persistent organic pollutants (POPs)	0	0	?	0	0	+	0	0
Urbanization and its impacts	+++	++	+	++	++	++	++	++

Sustainability, health, and well-being

There is growing discussion of the need to achieve sustainable environmental and social conditions. Achieving sustainability means not passing critical thresholds that would cause irreversible and detrimental changes such as the permanent collapse of major fisheries, melting of large polar ice-sheets (raising sea-levels several metres), or collapse of a state due to social disorder and violence. In other words, sustainability is about maintaining the ecological systems and processes upon which healthy life depends. Relatedly, the attainment of what has been called a balanced 'triple bottom line' (i.e. optimizing economic, social, and environmental conditions) should be seen as a *means*, not an *end*. The rationale for a high-grade 'triple bottom-line' is to enhance human experience, including health and survival.

Long-term thinking and planning for planetary well-being form the true bottom-line of 'sustainability', with health of humans, but also of other species, as the main criterion.

Sustainability will require us to achieve societies able to maintain, and live within the limits of, the natural resource base, and its ecosystems, and to maintain internal social cohesion. As noted earlier, humankind is now overloading the biosphere. One very helpful way of visualizing and thinking about this is in relation to our transgressing of critical 'planetary boundaries' (Rockstrom et al. 2009).

The restoration of balance, at global level, between human numbers, demands, waste generation, and the capacity of the planet to supply, replenish, and absorb is a huge and worldwide task – of a scale and type not previously undertaken by humankind. It will require great effort and imagination across all levels of society, and across all cultures (notwithstanding the historical fact that industrializing and erstwhile empire-building 'western' society has largely set this planetary overload process in motion). The task is far too big, complex, and electorally threatening to be undertaken by governments alone.

Figure 13.7 illustrates the scientific estimates of the number of humans that Earth can sustain at our current levels of consumption and waste generation. Most such estimates put Earth's human carrying-capacity limit at or below 8 billion people.

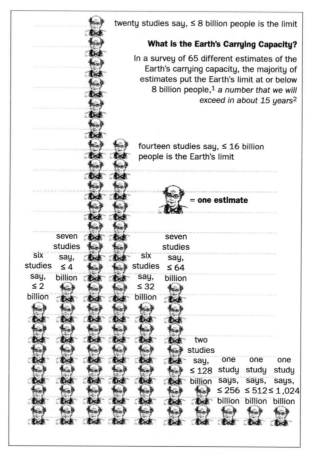

Figure 13.7 Estimates of the human overloading of the Earth's biocapacity

Source: UNEP-GEAS (2012)

There are now many ways to calculate your individual impact on the planet. If you have access to the Internet, go to one or two of the *Ecological Footprint* websites below. If you do a web search on 'ecological footprint' you will find similar sites for estimating personal footprints. Estimate your personal footprint size.

- http://www.myfootprint.org
- http://www.footprintnetwork.org/en/index.php/GFN/page/footprint_basics_overview/
- http://footprint.wwf.org.uk

Estimating your ecological footprint is one way to work out your impact on the planet, but you also need specific help on how to make the changes necessary.

Now, thinking of one of our most critical resources, let us look at your water use. Many countries now have advice lines to help you calculate your water consumption and to work out a way to reduce your water use. As we have seen earlier in the chapter, as climate change impacts increase, water conservation will be important even in current water-rich areas of the world. One site to help you calculate your water use is:

- http://www.home-water-works.org/calculator

Many water companies also have their own calculators. Here is one from Australia:

- http://www.yvwwatercalculator.com.au

Feedback

Your footprint size can be calculated in around ten minutes. The result tells you how many Earths would be needed if all 7 billion humans had a lifestyle like yours.

How much of 'nature' does your lifestyle require? These Ecological Footprint Questionnaires estimate how much productive land and water you need to support what you use and discard. How did you do? And how do the questionnaires compare? You will have seen that different websites ask very different questions and these influence your calculated footprint.

Your water use is also a good measure to take. Compare your water use with the WHO daily guidelines of 60 litres per person per day.

Summary

Globalization has become a reality of the twenty-first century, and – given current human numbers, ongoing population growth, and the extensification and intensification of economic activity (much of it based, seemingly inextricably, on fossil fuel combustion), global environmental changes are another entrenched reality of today and the immediate future. It is important to monitor global environmental change and its impacts on health and to relate estimates of health risks more directly to policy and social decision-making. This should be done globally, regionally, nationally, and locally. In 2013 at the UN climate change negotiations in Warsaw, the meeting saw an unprecedented hunger strike by the Philippines' representative Minister, and a mass walk-out by all the non-governmental organizations present. Speaking for the NGOs, Friends of the Earth stated, 'This Warsaw summit is achieving nothing to help protect vulnerable and poor communities or to reduce global carbon pollution – we must all do more in the months ahead to make the world wake up to the need for urgent action.' Christiana Figueres, Executive Secretary of the UN Framework Convention on Climate Change (UNFCCC), said: 'We have seen essential progress. But let us again be clear that we are witnessing ever more frequent, extreme weather events, and the poor and vulnerable are already paying the price.'

You have seen how the impacts of global environmental change are complex, they affect the climate, agricultural production, water, biodiversity and the atmosphere, each of which in turn has an impact on health. Scientific opinion points clearly to an urgent need to address the sustainability of global changes currently taking place, while public health research to identify current and future health risks from global environmental change remains challenging.

References

Alves, R. and Rosa, I. (2007) Biodiversity, traditional medicine and public health: where do they meet?, *Journal of Ethnobiology and Ethnomedicine*, 3(1): 14.

Campbell–Lendrum, D. and Corvalan, C. (2007) Climate change and developing-country cities: implications for environmental health and equity, *Journal of Urban Health*, 84 (3 suppl.): i109–i117.

Cline, W.R. (2007) *Global Warming and Agriculture: Impact Estimates by Country*. Washington, DC: Peterson Institute.

Cohen, J.E. (1995) Population growth and earth's human carrying capacity, *Science*, 269 (5222): 341–6.

Grundmann, R. (2006) Ozone and climate: scientific consensus and leadership, Science, *Technology and Human Values*, 31 (1): 73–101.

Lawler, J.J. (2009) Climate change adaptation strategies for resource management and conservation planning, *Annals of the New York Academy of Sciences*, 1162: 79–98.

Martens, P. (2009) Climate change and health, *Nederlands Tijdschrift voor Geneeskunde*, 153: A1420.

McIntyre, K.M., Setzkorn, C., Baylis, M., Waret-Szkuta, A., Caminade, C., Morse, A.P. et al. (2010) Impact of climate change on human and animal health, *Veterinary Record*, 167 (15): 586.

McMichael, A. (2005) Global environmental changes, climate change and human health, in K. Lee and J. Collin (eds.) *Global Change and Health*, pp. 126–46. Maidenhead: Open University Press.

Millar, C.I., Stephenson, N.L. and Stephens, S.L. (2007) Climate change and forests of the future: managing in the face of uncertainty, *Ecological Applications*, 17 (8): 2145–51.

Millennium Assessment Report (2000) *Graphic resources* [http://www.millenniumassessment.org/en/GraphicResources.aspx].

Myers, N., Mittermeier, R.A., Mittermeier, C.G., da Fonseca, G.A. and Kent, J. (2000) Biodiversity hotspots for conservation priorities, *Nature*, 403 (6772): 853–8.

Parr, M.J., Bennun, L., Boucher, T., Brooks, T., Chutas, C.A., Dinerstein, E. et al. (2009) Why we should aim for zero extinction, *Trends in Ecology and Evolution*, 24 (4): 181; author reply 183–4.

Rockstrom, J., Steffen, W., and Noone, K. (2009) A safe operating space for humanity, *Nature*, 461: 472–5.

Rudd, M.A. (2011) Scientists' opinions on the global status and management of biological diversity, *Conservation Biology*, 25 (6): 1165–75.

Stephens, C. (2012) Biodiversity and global health: hubris, humility and the unknown, *Environmental Research Letters*, 7 (1): 011008.

Stocker, T.F., Qin, D., Plattner, G.-K., Tignor, M.M.B., Allen, S.K., Nauels, A. et al. (eds) (2013) *Climate Change 2013: The Physical Science Basis. Contribution of Working Group I to the Fifth Assessment Report of the Intergovernmental Panel on Climate Change*. Cambridge: Cambridge University Press.

UNEP-GEAS (2012) One planet, how many people? A review of Earth's carrying capacity. Discussion Paper for the Year of Rio+20 [http://na.unep.net/geas/archive/pdfs/GEAS_Jun_12_Carrying_Capacity.pdf].

UNEP-WCMC (2011) *Health and Well Being of Communities Directly Dependent on Ecosystem Goods and Services: An Indicator for the Convention on Biological Diversity*. Cambridge: UNEP-World Conservation Monitoring Centre.

WRI (2013) *Per Capita CO$_2$ Emissions for Select Major Emitters, 2007 and 2030* (projected). Washington, DC: World Resources Institute [http://www.wri.org/resources/charts-graphs/capita-co2-emissions-select-major-emitters-2007-and-2030-projected].

WRI/UNDP/World Bank (World Resources Institute, in collaboration with the United Nations Development Programme and World Bank) (2005) *The Wealth of the Poor: Managing Ecosystems to Fight Poverty*. Washington, DC: World Resources Institute.

14 Global health and security

Preslava Stoeva

Overview

In this chapter, we will critically examine the links between global health issues and the field of security. We begin with an introduction to the concept of security, and the key debates surrounding how security is defined before exploring the links between global health and security by examining the specific examples of bioterrorism, emerging and re-emerging infectious diseases, and HIV/AIDS.

Learning objectives

After working through this chapter, you will be able to:

- define the concepts of national, international, and human security
- review trends towards a broadening of the security agenda
- identify three criteria for defining global health issues as security issues
- recognize why biological weapons, emerging and re-emerging infectious diseases, and HIV/AIDS have received attention from the security community
- understand the benefits and risks of linking global health with a security agenda

Key terms

Global health security: The set of issues arising out of the overlap between global health and national security concerns, including infectious disease epidemics and bioterrorism.

Human security: A concern with individual life and human dignity, involving safety from such chronic threats as hunger, disease, and repression, and protection from sudden and hurtful disruptions in the patterns of daily life (UNDP 1994: 22–3).

National security: The defence of the state against military and other types of serious threats to the state's sovereignty and survival.

Defining security

Security has been characterized as an 'essentially contested concept' (Buzan 1991) and an 'ambiguous symbol' (Wolfers 1952). Scholars of security studies and practitioners within the security policy community have offered a multitude of definitions over the years, but none has achieved widespread recognition. Disagreements cover various aspects of the term 'security', including the nature and scope of security (what is security?), the referent object of security (security for whom?), the nature of threats to security (security from what?), and the policies and resources needed to achieve security (how is security to be achieved?).

What is security?

Walter Lippmann, talking on the subject of US foreign policy in 1943 stated:

> A nation [state] is secure to the extent to which it is not in danger of having to sacrifice core values if it wishes to avoid war, and is able, if challenged, to maintain them by victory in such a war.

This definition places the interests of the nation-state, its protection, and the promotion of its vital interests at the heart of concept of security. The pursuit of security, according to Lippmann, requires military means, which need to exceed in relative terms those of an opponent or challenger of state security.

Barry Buzan argues that the discussion of security centres on the pursuit of *freedom from threat*, and adds that 'security is primarily about the fate of human collectivities, and only secondarily about the personal security of individual human beings' (Buzan 1991: 19). Buzan's work has had a profound impact on contemporary security debates, as he proposed the widening of the concept of security beyond military factors. He argued that the security of human collectivities was influenced by five categories of factors: military, political, economic, societal, and environmental.

Ken Booth takes debates over the nature and scope of security even further by contending that 'national and statist orthodoxies, which promote the idea of security *against* others' need to be re-conceptualized so as to 'conceive security as an instrumental value concerned to promote security *reciprocally*, as part of the invention of a more inclusive humanity' (Booth 2007: 2). Booth sees security not as a goal of foreign policy, or a pre-existing political condition, but as a *value* and as the *availability of choice*. He argues that people feel secure when they feel they can make choices in their daily lives – a view radically different from traditional conceptualizations of security.

The work of both Buzan and Booth signifies important post-Cold War developments in security thinking, which have opened the field, albeit in different ways, to allow concerns over public health to be considered in strategic terms as threats to security.

Security for whom?

The definitions of security provided above hint at the disagreements regarding the *object of security*, namely, the answer to the question 'security for whom?'. Traditional theories of security, including studies of national security, strategic studies and realist, neo-realist and some constructivist security scholars, envisaged the state as the primary object of security. They argue that the security of the state is a precondition for the security of its inhabitants. The state is a sovereign, territorially based political unit, characterized by central decision-making and hierarchical power structure, as discussed in Chapters 4 and 5. The assumption that the state is the primary object of security determines the scope and magnitude of security threats that are considered significant for policy-makers. When security is considered in state-centric terms, health concerns only matter if they affect large parts of the population, are defined by urgency, or present new and

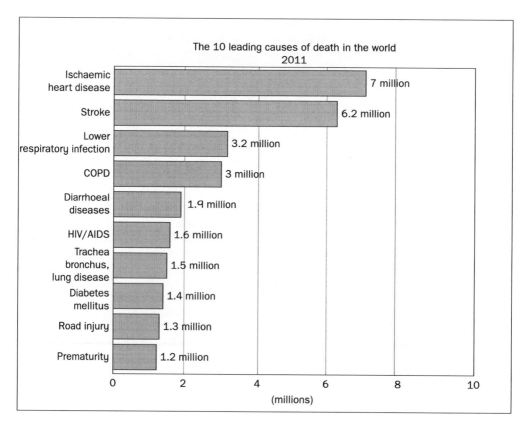

Figure 14.1 The ten leading causes of death in the world, 2011

Source: WHO Media Centre [http://who.int/mediacentre/factsheets/fs310/en/]

pressing challenges (e.g. new strands of the flu virus, multi-drug resistant strands of tuberculosis).

In the post-Cold War context of increasing internal conflicts and a diminishing number of state-to-state wars, some scholars have proposed a move away from the state as the object of security to a focus on the *individual* as an object of security. They have argued that *individual* insecurity – caused by ethnic tensions, poverty, economic insecurity, resource scarcity, etc. – drives state instability and global insecurity (see Brainard and Chollet 2007; Collier 2008; Duffield 2007; Kaldor 2007; Klare and Chandrani 1998). Ken Booth contends that we live in 'a world that is not working for most of its inhabitants' (2007: 12–13), as illustrated by the annual reports of the United Nations Development Programme. He argues that 'ordinary insecurities determine lives' (2007: 103), rather than big strategic threats. Some empirical evidence from the World Health Organization supports this view: the ten most common causes of death across the world are communicable and non-communicable diseases, rather than political conflict or violence (Figure 14.1). This figure illustrates how diseases pose an *existential threat* to individuals, which is the ultimate security threat.

Buzan, however, opposes the view that individual security should be a consideration in security studies. He argues that this may be counter-productive for the purposes of analysis and policy-making, because security cannot be complete for any individual . . . Most threats to individuals arise from the fact that people find themselves embedded in a human environment, which generates unavoidable social, economic and political pressures.

(Buzan 1991: 36–7)

Buzan envisages a permanent tension between the individual and the collective, where the needs of the whole are larger and more important than those of the unit.

Security from what?

Defining the concept and object of security is central to identifying specific security threats, which in turn is the basis on which to decide on policy priorities and the distribution of resources to address security threats. Security budgets tend to be generous and relatively stable over time (even in times of crisis), because security is the strategic priority of states. Policy communities may therefore be willing to characterize issues as security-related to gain political attention and access to resources. Identifying what security threats are relevant to a state is usually part of the process of formulating national security policy, which is a government responsibility. Security threats are also discussed by non-governmental organizations and academic and research communities, which attempt to project future threats that have the potential to disrupt the social, economic, and political life both within and outside states.

While traditional security scholars argue that threats stem from outside of the state and are military in nature, many studies published after the end of the Cold War sought to demonstrate empirically that conflicts and insecurity were caused by factors other than states' strategic considerations. These included military threats from non-state actors, ethnic or cultural identities, environmental degradation, resource scarcity/abundance, violations of human rights, transnational crime, poverty, underdevelopment, international trade, migration, and so on (e.g. Brainard and Chollet 2007; Collier 2008; Duffield 2007; Hough 2008; Kaldor 2007; Klare 2008; Klare and Chandrani 1998; Terriff et al. 1999). It is within this context of broadening the spectrum of security threats that scholars have argued that threats to human health should be on the security agenda, as will be discussed later on in the chapter.

How to achieve security?

The question about how security could be achieved is closely related to the previous three questions about the definition of security, the referent objects of security, and the nature of relevant security threats. For example, what threats are envisaged as important can give us some idea of the means needed to achieve security. Since traditional security threats were seen to stem from other states and their military capabilities, strategies were fairly simple – to seek allies and invest in the increase and development of military technologies. After the end of the Cold War, however, the number of conflicts taking place within states grew and the warring parties relied more heavily on small arms and light weapons. The question of how to achieve security became more challenging. In its Security Strategy, the Council of the European Union (2003) argued that conflicts can be diffused and avoided altogether, and security enhanced by facilitating economic development, growth, and better governance, instead of using traditional military methods (which continues to be the preferred approach of the United States).

In summary, there are four fundamental questions that define the field of security studies: the concept of security, the object of security, the nature of security threats, and the resources and methods to address these. Answers to these questions are interrelated and inter-dependent and help us formulate the working assumptions of our chosen approach to security. The nature of security threats has been contested and while traditionally they were seen primarily as military in nature, many scholars argue that other types of threats are also relevant. Let us now consider three main approaches to security in closer detail: national security, international/world security, and human security.

Activity 14.1

Based on the four questions discussed above: (i) what is security?, (ii) security for whom?, (iii) security from what?, and (iv) how to achieve security? – think about how you would argue that a health issue of your choice is a security problem. Now try making the opposite argument.

Feedback

Making an argument that a selected disease is a security issue requires you to think about how security is to be defined, about whether security should be centred on the state or the individual, and what exactly it is about the disease that you have chosen that threatens your selected object of security.

National security

National security as a concept has dominated security studies and studies of inter-state politics since the end of the Second World War. It refers to the security of the nation or the state. National security is a strategic priority of national governments, because, it is argued, without the survival of the state, no other priorities or goals of government can be achieved. Governments seek to protect and promote their national security through their military, economic, domestic, and foreign policies.

During the Cold War era, when tensions between the United States and the Soviet Union defined international relations, national security policies focused predominantly on external military threats, the accumulation of military power, and engaging in strategic alliances. This perspective, known as the *realist* (or *realpolitik*) approach, assumes that international relations are defined by conflict and states competing for power. The nuclear arms race between the two superpowers is a clear example of both sides seeking to enhance their security by building up a formidable arsenal.

While military and economic threats remain a core component of national security in post-Cold War politics, other issues such as mass migrations, environmental degradation, and acute epidemic infections are now considered possible threats to state security. Many of these 'new security threats' are transnational in character, where either the cause or effect, or both, transcend national borders. These transnational threats pose new challenges for states seeking to secure national interests, because states need to find ways to cooperate in order to achieve common goals.

Human security

Unlike national security, human security places the individual at the heart of security politics. Three competing conceptualizations of human security are at the heart of contemporary debates. These developed in the 1990s, building on liberal and social justice traditions and the politics of protection and promotion of universal human rights. Two of the conceptualizations are narrower in scope – the first is premised on the principles of natural rights and basic individual rights, which are to be protected and promoted by the international community (Alston 1992; Lauren 1998). The second conceptualization stems from the principles of humanitarian law, which require the protection of civilians and non-combatants in times of conflict, the safeguarding against genocide and war crimes, and the abolition of weapons of mass destruction, which may maim or kill indiscriminately (Boutros-Ghali 1992; Kaldor 2007; Mack 2005). This humanitarian conceptualization of human security aligns well with another core concept of contemporary security politics – the *Responsibility to Protect* (R2P). R2P emerged in response to the millions of victims of political violence in the twentieth century when some 262 million people were estimated killed by their own governments, including the humanitarian disasters of Rwanda, the former Yugoslavia, and East Timor.

The third conceptualization of human security represents a broader view and was introduced in the *Human Development Report* published annually by the United Nations Development Programme. In 1994, the report entitled 'New Dimensions of Human Security' argued that:

> The concept of security has for too long been interpreted narrowly: as security of territory from external aggression, or as protection of national interests in foreign policy, or as global security from the threat of nuclear holocaust . . . Forgotten were the legitimate concerns of ordinary people who sought security in their daily lives. For many of them, security symbolized protection from the threat of disease, hunger, unemployment, crime, social conflict, political repression and environmental hazards.

Human security was defined as 'freedom from fear and freedom from want', where freedom from fear referred to individual security from the threat of violence, while freedom from want represented the aspiration that people should be free from poverty and destitution and entitled to basic means of survival.

New Dimensions of Human Security (UNDP 1994) identified seven areas of human security – economic security, food security, health security, environmental security, personal security, community security, and political security. Human security is seen as universal, its components interdependent, much like universal human rights. This way of thinking about human security, however, has drawn criticisms regarding the manageability of the concept, its practicality, and the danger that it can turn into a potential laundry list of 'bad things that can happen' and lead to unnecessary securitization of issues (Krause 2007; Mack 2002, 2005; Owen 2004).

Many recognize the interdependence between human security and national security (Commission on Human Security 2003). When a state is insecure, it is very difficult for individuals within that state to remain secure. Similarly, state security is built upon the security of its individual citizens. When individuals are insecure, it becomes more difficult for the basic functions of the state to operate. But while such interdependence is logical in theory, practice presents us with important tensions – the continued dominance of national security perspectives, the discordance within the human security approach, and the different resources required in the pursuit of these approaches – primarily military in the case of national security, and multiple – including finance, expertise, investment, education, science, etc., required for the pursuit of broad human security.

 Activity 14.2

Read the following two definitions of security. For each definition, describe who the object of security is and provide three examples of a security threat defined in this way.

1 'In anarchy, security is the highest end. Only if survival is assured can states seek such other goals as tranquility, profit and power.' (Waltz 1979: 126)
2 'The "logic of security" should be broadened beyond territorial defence, national interests and nuclear deterrence to include "universal concerns" and the prevention of conflicts, but also crucially a cooperative global effort to eradicate poverty and underdevelopment.' (UNDP 1994: 22)

Feedback

1 For the first definition, the object of security is the state. Threats to the national security of a state might include a military attack, a sudden flood of refugees due to a conflict in a neighbouring state, or an economic crisis.
2 The object of security in the second definition is the individual. Threats to human security might include loss of employment, lack of basic needs such as food and water, or a local environmental disaster.

How is health related to security?

The 1994 UNDP Human Development Report identified poor health as a threat to human security, a position reaffirmed in the 2003 Report of the Commission on Human Security. Good health is 'essential' because illness, disability, and death are critical threats to human security. The Commission argued that violence, infectious diseases, and poverty are the three health challenges that critically impact human security (see Figure 14.2).

Perhaps more notable is the way in which health issues have come to be included in the traditional concerns of national security. Health has traditionally been deemed a 'low politics' issue, that is, a domestic concern of social policy unworthy of priority considera-tion in the 'high-politics' agenda occupied by strategic foreign defence and economic policy. Laurie Garrett's influential article 'The return of infectious diseases' (1996) and the Institute of Medicine's (IOM) Report for The National Academy (US) *America's Vital Interests in Global Health* (1997) mark a watershed in the attitude towards health. Both of these publications argued that emerging and re-emerging infectious diseases had poten-tially serious implications for national security. Health issues have steadily made their way onto national security agendas and strategic documents (Feldbaum et al. 2006). The concept of global health security is the area where national security and global health concerns meet.

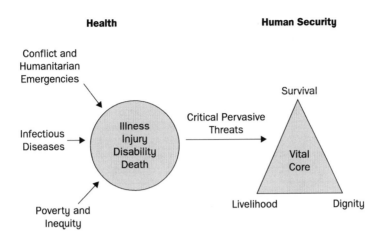

Figure 14.2 Health and human security linkages

Source: Based on Commission on Human Security (2003)

The overlap between the fields of public health, national and international security is highly contested. What issues constitute global health security threats is a critical question, as it challenges the notion that health issues pose an immediate threat to national security. A number of scholars are warning that expanding national security agendas to incorporate too many issues may not only be unproductive, but may actually be harmful to humanitarian politics and may impede health cooperation.

Clearly not all global health issues have been considered threats to national security. While no systematic criteria exist, the characteristics of health issues already under discussion help to identify some criteria.

- They pose a severe risk to social well-being by impacting population health status, the health status of a strategic group such as the armed forces, or the economy.
- They have an impact across borders and notably in strategically important countries.
- They pose an acute threat in a relatively immediate time-frame.

These attributes may help explain why some long-term health issues that cause high morbidity and mortality, such as chronic and non-communicable diseases, are not presently considered national security threats. Whose security is being considered is also an important determinant. To understand these criteria in greater detail, and in relation to specific health issues, the following sections will examine bioterrorism, emerging and re-emerging infectious diseases, and HIV/AIDS, which have been identified by many as the most potent threats to states' security interests.

Bioterrorism and biological weapons

The spectre of biological weapons represents the clearest link between health and national security policy. Biological warfare is the deliberate spread of disease among an adversary's population, livestock or plant life. Biological warfare involves the use of living organisms or the by-products of living organisms as instruments for waging conflict. The development of biological weapons based on these diseases is attractive to states and terrorist organizations because they:

- have the potential to cause mass casualties;
- can be made with materials and information that are widely available and commonly used in legitimate commercial activities;
- are significantly less expensive to produce and easier to conceal than a comparable nuclear programme.

The production and use of biological weapons are prohibited internationally by means of the Convention on the Prohibition of the Development, Production and Stockpiling of Bacteriological (Biological) and Toxin Weapons and on their Destruction (Biological Weapons Convention – BWC), which came into force in 1975. In 2013, the Convention had 170 state signatories (UNOG 2013).

Despite the international prohibition detailed in BWC, events during the mid-1990s brought biological weapons onto both the national security and global health agendas. In 1995, Iraqi defectors revealed a larger and more sophisticated biological weapons programme than previously known, including the production of *Bacillus anthracis* and the botulinum toxin (Henderson 1998). The 9/11 terrorist attacks on the World Trade Center in 2001 were followed by what became known as the anthrax attacks – five letters containing *Bacillus anthracis* were mailed to US government officials and media outlets. Twenty-two people developed anthrax, and five died as a result. Despite the relatively low number of deaths, the incident caused great disruption. Senate office buildings and postal facilities were closed, US mail irradiated, and 33,000 people required prophylaxis. These events led to large-scale efforts and collaboration between the public health and security communities to enhance domestic preparedness for the eventuality of a terrorist biological attack. The highest priority bioterrorism agents, according to the US Centers for Disease Control and Prevention, are those that pose a risk to national security because they:

- can be easily disseminated or transmitted from person to person;
- result in high mortality rates and have the potential for major public health impact;
- might cause public panic and social disruption; and
- require special action for public health preparedness.

These agents are:

- anthrax (*Bacillus anthracis*);
- botulism (*Clostridium botulinum* toxin);
- plague (*Yersinia pestis*);
- smallpox (*Variola major*);
- tularemia (*Francisella tularensis*);
- viral haemorrhagic fevers – filoviruses (e.g. ebola, marburg) and arenaviruses (e.g. lassa, machupo]).

The development and proliferation of biological weapons are a transnational problem, which poses a considerable challenge for both the health and security communities. Denying access to such weapons to rogue states and non-state actors is a global priority.

Emerging and re-emerging infectious diseases

> In the context of infectious diseases, there is nowhere in the world from which we are
> remote and no one from whom we are disconnected.
>
> (US Institute of Medicine 1992)

The last 30 years have witnessed the emergence of new and the resurgence of old
diseases, some increasingly resistant to antimicrobials and other drug treatments. At
least thirty new diseases have been identified since 1973. Previously known diseases
such as cholera, yellow fever, and dengue have re-emerged dramatically, while tuberculosis has re-emerged in a multi-drug-resistant form. Disease vectors have also become
resistant to insecticides and increased their geographic range, bringing malaria, African
sleeping sickness, West Nile virus, Rift Valley fever, yellow fever, and dengue into new
areas and onto new continents.

Emerging and re-emerging infectious diseases (ERIDs) were not generally viewed as
threats to national security until the 1990s. In 2000, the US National Intelligence Council
(NIC) published *The Global Infectious Disease Threat and its Implications for the United
States*, an unprecedented evaluation of global health issues by the American national
security community. The report considers ERIDs a threat to US and global security
because it argues diseases will 'endanger US citizens at home and abroad, threaten US
armed forces deployed overseas, and exacerbate social and political instability in key
countries and regions in which the United States has significant interests' (US National
Intelligence Council 2000). The National Intelligence Council (NIC) report is considered
exceptional because it effectively expanded the definition of national security to include
threats from selected infections. The NIC report, much like the majority of the health
security literature, continues to be state-centric, namely, to view politics at the level of the
state. Its focus is on impacts large enough to affect the national political and economic
interests of states, as well as regional and international stability.

The policy response to ERIDs involves support for similar measures as those for identifying and responding to bioterrorism, in particular a strong global disease surveillance
and monitoring system, backed by reliance on public health systems. A number of mechanisms have been put into place to improve global responses to naturally occurring and
deliberately caused disease outbreaks. The Global Outbreak Alert and Response Network
and the revised International Health Regulations (WHO 2005) are two such mechanisms.

HIV/AIDS

In 2000, an unprecedented UN Security Council (UNSC) meeting was held on the impact of
HIV/AIDS on peace and security in Africa. This was the first time that the UNSC, a body
charged with the maintenance of international peace and security, had examined a health
issue as a relevant concern. The United States Security Council Ambassador at the time,
Richard Holbrooke, argued that it was the cruellest irony to send peacekeepers to stop
conflict during which they unintentionally spread HIV. In July 2000, the UNSC passed
Resolution 1308 requiring further training of peacekeepers on preventing the spread of HIV
and AIDS, and encouraging UN member states to increase HIV prevention, testing, and
treatment for those deployed on peacekeeping missions. The resolution resulted in a UN
training programme to disseminate information about HIV and the creation of a new UNAIDS
Office on AIDS, Security and Humanitarian Response. Perhaps more important than the
resolution itself was the discussion of HIV/AIDS at the highest international security forum.

The HIV/AIDS epidemic has been characterized as a security threat for three main reasons: the speed with which it had spread since the 1980s when it was first discovered; the high mortality, which many believed would undermine economic development and societal stability in already poor countries, causing state failure; and its effects on international peacekeeping (McInnes 2006). Over the last two decades, concerns were raised that HIV/AIDS would destabilize nations beyond sub-Saharan Africa that were critical to American strategic interests and global stability. The nations typically included in this group were India, China, and Russia. The campaign linking HIV/AIDS and security has lost some momentum in recent years. Scenarios of failing states and decimated populations that were projected at the start of the twenty-first century did not materialize and with the increased availability and accessibility of anti-retroviral therapies (ARTs), supported by both public and private funding, people infected with the virus have gained near normal life expectancy.

✎ **Activity 14.3**

Think about the arguments used to link the HIV/AIDS pandemic to national security concerns. Choose another global public health issue and apply the three criteria discussed above (speed, mortality, and impact on peacekeeping). Does it:

- pose a severe risk to social well-being by impacting population health status, the health status of a strategic group such as the armed forces, or the economy?
- have an impact across borders and notably in strategically important countries?
- pose an acute threat in a relatively immediate time-frame?

Write a one-page letter to the editor of a health journal arguing why your global health issue is or is not a national security threat.

Feedback

Some interesting global public health issues you might wish to test are non-communicable diseases, the global obesity epidemic, neglected tropical diseases, lack of access by the poor to essential drugs, or the health consequences of global environmental change. Some satisfy two of the three criteria. Depending on its nature, global environmental change may satisfy all three criteria.

Risks and benefits of linking health and security

The recent characterization of global health issues as security threats has resulted in greater political attention and funding to address some infectious diseases and bioterrorism. This attention has allowed considerable scaling up of some global health activities and initiatives. In recent years, however, there has been growing scepticism regarding the causal links between health and security. The long-term implications of global health's move into the areas of security and high politics remain unclear.

Observers from the fields of security and health have criticized viewing infectious diseases through the lens of security. Objections within the security community concern the overly broad definition of security. A common refrain is that 'if everything is a security issue, then nothing is'. It is also argued that the link between health and security is speculative, too indirect, and inappropriately concerned with non-military threats. There are further anxieties about the ethics and impact on vulnerable groups of presenting ill health as a security concern. The public health and development aid communities have challenged the securitization of health for making global health activities subservient to political priorities and narrow national interests, and turning them into a tool for the pursuit of foreign policy objectives. There are growing concerns among the global health community regarding the limited attention paid to the causes and consequences of non-communicable diseases, which are now prevalent as much in the Global North as in the Global South.

The development of a better understanding of the linkages between global health and security politics and of the implications for both health and security require scholars and practitioners on both sides to engage in a more effective dialogue. Such dialogue needs to be inter-disciplinary and sensitive to the needs of people across the world. The global health community needs to carefully carve its role in world affairs, so as not to be overshadowed, intentionally or unintentionally, by the work of other policy communities.

✏ Activity 14.4

Consider once again the global public health issue selected in Activity 14.3. Are there advantages or disadvantages to health in addressing this issue as a threat to national security? What positive or negative effects do you think the security community could experience in incorporating selected health problems into its agenda?

Feedback

In considering the above, you will need to think about what different goals and perspectives the health and security communities might have, as well as their different degrees of influence over the political agenda. The health community might benefit from the raising of selected health issues higher on the public policy agenda. However, this might be at the expense of skewing the agenda and thus neglecting other, equally pressing health needs. The security community could benefit from dealing in a timely and appropriate manner with a real threat to a population's well-being. However, it may also be seen as risking the opening up of the security agenda too broadly.

Summary

In this chapter, you have learnt about the recent linking of health and security by various scholarly and policy communities, which has arisen amid recognition of the global nature of certain health issues, notably infectious diseases and bioterrorism. This should have encouraged you to be more critical in reflecting on the relevance and appropriateness of placing health and security in close proximity.

References

Alston, P. (ed.) (1992) *The United Nations and Human Rights: A Critical Appraisal.* Oxford: Oxford University Press.

Booth, K. (2007) *Theory of World Security.* Cambridge: Cambridge University Press.

Boutros-Ghali, B. (1992) *An Agenda for Peace: Preventive Diplomacy, Peacemaking and Peacekeeping.* New York: United Nations.

Brainard, L. and Chollet, D. (eds) (2007) *Too Poor for Peace? Global Poverty, Conflict, and Security in the 21st Century.* Washington, DC: Brookings Institution Press.

Buzan, B. (1991) *People, States and Fear: An Agenda for International Security Studies in the Post-Cold War Era* (2nd edn). London: Harvester Wheatsheaf.

Collier, P. (2008) *The Bottom Billion: Why the Poorest Countries Are Failing and What Can Be Done About It.* Oxford: Oxford University Press.

Commission on Human Security (2003) *Human Security Now.* New York: Commission on Human Security.

Council of the European Union (2003) *A Secure Europe in a Better World*, Brussels, 12 December 2003 [http://www.consilium.europa.eu/uedocs/cmsUpload/78367.pdf; last accessed 12 November 2013].

Duffield, M. (2007) *Development, Security and Unending War.* Cambridge: Polity Press.

Evans, J. (2010) Pandemics and national security, *Global Security Studies*, 1: 100–9.

Feldbaum, H., Patel, P., Sondorp, E. and Lee, K. (2006) Global health and national security: the need for critical engagement, *Medicine, Conflict and Survival*, 22: 192–8.

Garrett, L. (1996) The return of infectious disease, *Foreign Affairs*, 75: 66–79.

Henderson, D.A. (1998) Bioterrorism as a public health threat, *Emerging Infectious Diseases*, 4 (3): 488–92.

Hough, P. (2008) *Understanding Global Security* (2nd edn). London: Routledge.

Institute of Medicine (1992) *Emerging Infections: Microbial Threats to Health in the United States.* Committee on Emerging Microbial Threats to Health. Washington, DC: National Academy Press.

Institute of Medicine (1997) *America's Vital Interest in Global Health: Protecting Our People, Enhancing Our Economy, and Advancing Our International Interests.* Washington, DC: National Academies Press [http://www.nap.edu/openbook.php?record_id=5717; accessed 25 July 2013].

Kaldor, M. (2007) *Human Security: Reflections on Globalization and Intervention.* Cambridge: Polity Press.

Klare, M. (2008) *Rising Powers, Shrinking Planet: How Scarce Energy Is Creating a New World Order.* New York: Metropolitan Books.

Klare, M. and Chandrani, Y. (eds) (1998) *World Security: Challenges for a New Century* (3rd edn). New York: St. Martin's Press.

Krause, K. (2007) Towards a practical human security agenda. Policy Paper No. 26. Geneva: Geneva Centre for the Democratic Control of Armed Forces [http://www.dcaf.ch/Publications/Towards-a-Practical-Human-Security-Agenda; accessed 8 November 2013].

Lauren, P. (1998) *The Evolution of Human International Rights: Visions Seen.* University Park, PA: Pennsylvania State University Press.

Lippmann, W. (1943) *US Foreign Policy: Shield of the Republic.* Boston, MA: Little, Brown.

Mack, A. (2002) *A Report on the Feasibility of Creating an Annual Human Security Report.* Cambridge, MA: Program on Humanitarian Policy and Conflict Research, Harvard University.

Mack, A. (2005) *Human Security Report 2005: War and Peace in the 21st Century.* New York: Oxford University Press.

McInnes, C. (2006) HIV/AIDS and security, *International Affairs*, 82: 315–26.

Owen, T. (2004) Human security – conflict, critique and consensus: colloquium remarks and a proposal for a threshold-based definition, *Security Dialogue*, 35: 373–87.

Terriff, T., Croft, S., James, L. and Morgan, P. (1999) *Security Studies Today.* Cambridge: Polity Press.

United Nations Development Programme (1994) *Human Development Report 1994: New Dimensions of Human Security.* Oxford: Oxford University Press.

UNOG (2013) *Disarmament* [http://www.unog.ch/80256EE600585943/(httpPages)/7BE6CBBEA0477B52 C12571860035FD5C?OpenDocument; accessed 25 April 2014].

US National Intelligence Council (2000) National Intelligence estimate: the global infectious disease threat and its implications for the United States, *Environmental Change and Security Project Report*, 6: 33–65.

Waltz, K.N. (1979) *Theory of International Politics*. New York: McGraw-Hill.

WHO (2005) *International Health Regulations* (2nd edn). Geneva: World Health Organization.

Wolfers, A. (1952) 'National security' as an ambiguous symbol, *Political Science Quarterly*, 67 (4): 481–502.

Postscript: Ebola

As this book went to press, the outbreak of Ebola virus in West Africa gathered pace, causing great loss of human life and a major international response. It is hard to predict the long-term impact of the current outbreak beyond the immediate human tragedy of many lives lost where systems have been overwhelmed and unable to respond. At the same time, even as the crisis is still unfolding, the great relevance to the issues explored in this book is evident.

First, the current outbreak of Ebola underlines the interconnectedness between people in different areas in the globe. It emphasises that health issues regardless of where they occur can very quickly become global. The fact that the original outbreak happened in the border area of Guinea, Sierra Leone and Liberia, where the population is highly mobile is thought to have contributed to the spread. Cases in North America and Europe occurred as a result of people travelling or being repatriated. Governments in Europe and the US have justified intervention and support to countries in West Africa not simply on humanitarian grounds, but by saying that preventing an outbreak at home will require controlling it abroad.

Second, the different risks faced by people depending on where they live and their personal circumstances highlights the impact of social inequalities on health outcomes. Peter Piot, discoverer of the Ebola virus, has referred to the circumstances in West Africa – that of poverty combined with post-conflict societies alongside weak and underfunded health systems – as a 'perfect storm' for Ebola, while countries with greater resources and stronger health systems are able to control disease outbreaks more quickly.

Third, reactions to the outbreak have been diverse, with some countries closing borders and airlines suspending flights to affected areas. In the beginning responses to Ebola were led by one non-governmental organisation – Medicins Sans Frontieres (MSF) and WHO has come under criticism for an initially slow and ineffective response. This will likely have a bearing on the discussions of the organisation's reform in the future. Following the initial lack of action, the international response and solidarity has increased with the US, the UK and France amongst others contributing resources and manpower.

Fourth, Ebola and responses to the current outbreak have put health security firmly back on the agenda. In September 2014 the UN Security Council passed a resolution on Ebola, the first time such a resolution has ever been passed on a disease. In addition, support to affected countries by the US has largely been led by the military, very much framing Ebola as a security as much as a health issue.

These are just some ways in which the current outbreak is likely to affect and be affected by the issues discussed in this book; highlighting the pace of change in global governance of health. Above all it shows how important these issues are for the prevention of and responses to future health crises.

Autumn 2014

Index

Note: Key terms are in **bold** type.